74.00

MEDICAL
INTELLIGENCE
UNIT

ACUTE REJECTION OF LIVER GRAFTS

G. Gubernatis, M.D., Ph.D.

Medizinische Hochschule Hannover
Hannover, Germany

R.G. LANDES COMPANY
AUSTIN

Medical Intelligence Unit

ACUTE REJECTION OF LIVER GRAFTS

R.G. LANDES COMPANY
Austin / Georgetown

CRC Press is the exclusive worldwide distributor of publications of the Medical Intelligence Unit.
CRC Press, 2000 Corporate Blvd., NW, Boca Raton, FL 33431. Phone: 407/994-0555.

Submitted: February 1993
Published: May 1993

Production: Terry Nelson, Judith Kemper
Copy Editor: Constance Kerkaporta

Please address all inquiries to the Publisher:
R.G. Landes Company, 909 Pine Street, Georgetown, TX 78626
or
P.O. Box 4858, Austin, TX 78765
Phone: 512/ 863 7762 • FAX: 512/ 863 0081

While the authors, editors and publisher believe that drug selection and dosage and the specifications and usage of equipment and devices, as set forth in this book, are in accord with current recommendations and practice at the time of publication, they make no warranty, expressed or implied, with respect to material described in this book. In view of the ongoing research, equipment development, changes in governmental regulations and the rapid accumulation of information relating to the biomedical sciences, the reader is urged to carefully review and evaluate the information provided herein.

Library of Congress Cataloging-in-Publication Data
Gubernatis, G.
Acute Rejection of Liver Grafts, edited by G. Gubernatis
p. cm.—(Medical Intelligence Unit)
Includes bibliographical references and index.
ISBN 1-879702-64-9/CATALOG # LN0264 (hard) $89.95
1. Liver—Transplantation—Immunological aspects. 2. Graft rejection. 3. Liver—Biopsy, Needle.
I. Gubernatis, G. II. Series
[DNLM: 1. Liver Transplantation—immunology. 2. Graft Rejection. WI 770 A189 1993]
RD546.A28 1993
617.5'56—dc20

DNLM/DLC
for Library of Congress

93-15552
CIP

Acknowledgment

The experimental part of this study was supported by the Stiftung Volkswagenwerk, the clinical part by the Deutsche Forschungsgemeinschaft (DFG-Pi48).

In the experimental part a close cooperation with the Primate Center T.N.O. in Rijswijk/The Netherlands was the presupposition and the fruitful basis for the animal experiments. The whole study lasted for several years and many coworkers participated in these and previously done experiments. The main coworkers of the experimental work-group (besides the authors) were as follows:

Prof. Balner, previous director of T.N.O. Rijswijk
Prof. van Es, previous director of T.N.O. Rijswijk

Surgical part:
Prof. Dr. P. Neuhaus, Hannover/Berlin
Prof. Dr. W. Lauchart, Hannover/Tübingen
Dr. R. Viebahn, Hannover/Tübingen
Dr. G. Steinhoff, Hannover

Anesthesiological part:
Dr. A. Bornscheuer, Hannover

Immunological part including laboratory assistance:
Dr. M. Jonker, Rijswijk
Mrs. E. van der Linden, Rijswijk

Histopathological part:
PD Dr. F. J. Vonnahme, Hannover/Minden

Animal care and local organization:
Mr. H. Wirsema, Rijswijk

Engineering and organizational and surgical assistance:
Mr. W. Schüttler, Hannover

Technical and surgical assistants:
Mrs. H. Basse, Hannover/Oldenburg
Mrs. B. Wiehe, Hannover

The clinical part of this study was based on a detailed documentation system developed by the author together with Mr. G. Tusch under the assistance of Mrs. M. Mueller.

We are especially grateful to Mrs. S. Siegismund for the illustrations of the tables and figures and to Mrs. R. Drewitz for all the secretarial work.

CONTRIBUTORS

G. Gubernatis, Editor
Medizinische Hochschule Hannover

John J. Fung
Pittsburgh Transplantation Institute

J. Kemnitz
Essen
(formerly Medizinische Hochschule Hannover)

Ignazio Roberto Marino
Pittsburgh Transplantation Institute

Björn Nashan
Medizinische Hochschule Hannover

R. Pichlmayr
Medizinische Hochschule Hannover

Hans Jürgen Schlitt
Medizinische Hochschule Hannover

Thomas E. Starzl
Pittsburgh Transplantation Institute

CONTENTS

Early Postoperative Rejection After Liver Transplantation: An Experimental and Clinical Study

G. Gubernatis, J. Kemnitz, R. Pichlmayr

INTRODUCTION

Acute rejection is one of the most important problems in the transplantation of parenchymatous organs. This regards the frequency of rejection phenomena as well as the seriousness of its consequences. In general, the problem of "rejection" will exist as long as it is not possible to modify the recipient's immunological status to achieve tolerance. Presumably, this goal will not be achievable in the near future and immunosuppression will therefore be necessary to avert rejection. Increasing experience in the clinical management of immunosuppressive agents and the introduction of cyclosporin A as an essential part of immunosuppression have significantly improved results. Yet as various statistics generally demonstrate, the transplantation survival rates of kidneys could be improved by 20% and the recipient mortality could be decreased to low percentages. Nevertheless, maintaining the fine line between adequate suppression of rejection on the one hand and avoidance of toxicity and over-immunosuppression on the other is difficult. This requires prompt diagnosis and treatment of an acute rejection.

Immunologically the liver is a remarkable organ, especially in two respects:

1. Obviously, the liver is less sensitive to antibody-mediated immunoreactions. At least in the beginning of this study, hyperacute rejection after liver transplantation was not observed, neither in an animal model nor in the clinical situation.

2. The diagnosis of liver graft rejection is difficult. In contrast to kidney transplantation in which rejection can easily and clearly be diagnosed by both clinical and especially histological findings, the diagnosis of rejection of a liver graft causes serious problems. Pathognomonic histological signs of rejection, particularly regarding higher grades of rejection, do not exist. Furthermore,

during the first week it can be very difficult to distinguish nonimmunological causes of graft deterioration from immunological ones. Moreover, some immunological changes that appear similar to acute rejection are in fact completely reversible. At which stage a change should be considered rejection is a question of definition. The decisive question is at which stage such a finding requires treatment. Tolerating such a stage too long could reduce the effectiveness of treatment. On the other side treating such findings too early with highly toxic drugs unnecessarily puts the patient at risk.

The uncertainty in the consideration of histological findings corresponds to the difficulty in evaluating the significance of clinical signs. Neither deterioration of liver function tests nor general changes in the patient's con-

dition can be considered pathognomonic or typical for immunological or nonimmunological deteriorations.

The best possible diagnostic approach is therefore based on a combined assessment of clinical and histological findings.

The objectives of the study therefore were to determine the natural course of acute immunological rejection in the liver graft. These data should improve diagnostic and therapeutic decision-making. Moreover, the specific resistance of the liver graft to hyperacute rejection, i.e., to circulating antibodies, is considered.

Experimental and clinical studies were undertaken. In order to obtain results in the experimental part that were most relevant to the human situation, the Rhesus monkey was chosen as an animal model.

EARLY POSTOPERATIVE REJECTION AFTER LIVER TRANSPLANTATION

ANIMALS AND METHODS

Forty-seven orthotopic liver transplantations were performed on rhesus monkeys in the Primate Center of the T.N.O. in Rijswijk (The Netherlands).

1. ANIMALS

The monkeys (*Maccaca mulatta*) were either imported or they were bred in the Primate Center. All animals lived in the Primate Center for several years and could be observed continuously over a long period of time. Preexisting diseases and infections could therefore be excluded. At the time of operation the animals had a body weight ranging from 3.5 to 7.5 kg, most of them 4.5 to 5.5 kg. The donor-recipient pairs had a similar body weight.

2. STUDY GROUPS

Three different animal groups were used and four research groups were established from them:

I. ANIMALS WITH SPONTANEOUS COURSE

Twenty-four animals received no immunosuppression neither baseline nor for the treatment of rejection.

II. ANIMALS RECEIVING BASIC IMMUNOSUPPRESSION

Seventeen animals received basic immunosuppression, however, no additional rejection treatment was administered. Prednisolone 1 mg/kg body weight and cyclosporin A 10 mg/kg body weight given intramuscularly in a single dose were administered on a daily basis starting at the first postoperative day. The cyclosporin A dosage was reduced according to serum levels: a therapeutic range of 400-700 ng/ml (nonspecific polyclonal RIA in whole blood) was desired. Multiple measurements of the cyclosporin A level as well as assessment of renal function were used to determined toxicity. Each case was carefully documented with regard to the postoperative course.

III. COURSE AFTER CESSATION OF BASIC IMMUNOSUPPRESSION

In 10 animals basic immunosuppression was withheld during a period of well-being in order to provoke acute rejection. In three animals rejection was treated by using the monoclonal antibody FN18. This is an anti-CD3 receptor antibody. It was given for 10 days in a dosage of 1 mg/kg body weight for the first treatment period and 2 mg/kg body weight, whenever a second treatment period of 10 days was performed.

IV. DONOR SPECIFIC SENSITIZATION

In six animals donor specific sensitization was performed. In order to achieve specific sensitization, blood of the individual donor was subcutaneously injected into the recipient several times and skin was transplanted. The development of donor specific antibodies in the recipient was monitored. At the time of transplantation the lymphocytotoxic test was strongly positive in all cases.

3. PREOPERATIVE MANAGEMENT OF THE ANIMALS

For all animals complete RhLA typing including the DR-locus was available. For all donor recipient pairs a lymphocytotoxic test (cross match) was performed. Several days prior to operation the status of the animals was assessed again. This included blood sampling (red and white blood count, coagulation, liver enzymes, bilirubin, renal function). The day prior to operation the animals remained unfed with free access to water.

4. ANESTHESIA AND POSITIONING OF THE ANIMALS

As premedication and to begin anesthesia, ketamine hydrochloride 4 mg/kg body weight and acepromazine maleate 0.5-1 mg/kg body weight were administered intramuscularly. The animals were positioned in a foamy plastic bed. A heating pad was used in order to maintain the body temperature even during longer operations in a nearly normal range. After peripheral insertion of a cannula anesthesia was intensified by administering ketamine hydrochloride 2 mg/kg body weight intravenously. Then the animal was intubated and put on mechanical ventilation using a nitrous-oxide-oxygen mixture of 3:1. After insertion of a gastric tube, central catheters were inserted surgically into the vena jugularis interna and the arteria carotis on the right side. To maintain anesthesia 0.5-1 mg/kg body weight ketamine hydrochloride was administered every 1/2-1 hour. If anesthesia became too light 2 mg/kg body weight thiopental was administered additionally. There was no need for further relaxation. Ringers lactate was infused for fluid replacement. Intraoperative loss of fluid was replaced with Makrodex, human albumin or fresh blood derived from other animals. Systolic blood pressure was always maintained above 70 mmHg, the heart rate was below 130-140/min (normal frequency of the Rhesus monkey).

Further procedures in the donor:

Just prior to the perfusion of the organs with cold storage solution, blood was sampled from the arterial cannula. This blood could be transfused later into the recipient if necessary.

Further procedures in the recipient:

Cardiovascular changes caused by an elevated potassium level just after the reperfusion were avoided or reduced by administering calcium prior to and during reperfusion. Metabolic acidosis was compensated by administering sodium bicarbonate. Administration of catecholamines was never required. Anesthesia was maintained at a deep stage until the end of the operation to avoid reflex spasms, e.g., caused by suturing the peritoneum. In particular, laryngospasm occurred in previous series and were always dangerous. The animals were allowed to breath spontaneously when they had gained a temperature of at least 36°C. Extubation was performed after the animals regained sufficient respiration and reflexes. Then the cannulas were removed and the animals were put back into a warm cage.

A broad spectrum antibiotic was administered as perioperative prophylaxis.

5. OPERATIVE PROCEDURE

In general, both the donor and the recipient operation require particularly careful and skillful operative technique because of the very small and vulnerable structures involved. On the other hand, speed is required in order to avoid cooling of the animal and lengthy anesthesia. Such requirements could only be achieved by a standardization in every detail of the technique.

5.1 OPERATION OF THE DONOR ANIMAL

The operation of the donor animal can be divided into five phases:

I. INITIAL PREPARATION

After opening the abdomen through a median incision the liver is freed from adhesions. The left triangular ligament and the lesser omentum are transsected. The preparation of the hepatoduodenal ligament is started by the separation of the gastroduodenal artery, looping of the common bile duct, dissection of the portal vein and separation of the remaining lymph and nerve tissue close to the pancreas. Then the common hepatic artery and the celiac trunk are dissected up to the aorta. At this stage the splenic artery remains in situ. The infrahepatic vena cava is carefully dissected from the retroperitoneum and one or more veins branching to the suprarenal gland are separated. The infrahepatic part of the vena cava is looped. Then the liver is dissected completely on the right side from the retroperitoneum and the diaphragm. Then the omentum is dissected from right caudal to left cranial and the aorta is looped distally, close to the bifurcation.

The dissection of the small and large bowel is performed as the last step in order to avoid excessive lymph fluid floating from the dissection line to the hilus and right hepatic region, obscuring the operative field thereby making preparation of the small structures more difficult.

II. PREPARATION JUST PRIOR TO PERFUSION

After ligation and transsection of the common bile duct, sternotomy is performed. The pericardium is opened. Then cannulas for the perfusion are inserted into the abdominal aorta distally and the portal vein. The splenic artery is ligated and transsected.

III. PERFUSION

After clamping the ascending aorta and opening the inferior vena cava within the pericardium and at the level of the branching of the renal veins, perfusion via the aorta and portal vein starts simultaneously. In the present study Eurocollins solution was used. The gravity-fed perfusion simulated physiological pressures of about 120-150 cm H_2O for the aorta and 20 cm H_2O for the portal vein. A perfusion volume of 500 ml was used for both.

IV. REMOVAL OF THE LIVER

After removal of the perfusion cannulas the diaphragm is separated around the suprahepatic vena cava. The infrahepatic vena cava and the portal vein are transsected. The celiac trunk is removed together with a long segment of the thoracic aorta and the whole liver is removed and stored in cold solution.

V. DETAILED PREPARATION OF THE LIVER EX SITU

As a consequence of the procedure described above the liver is nearly completely prepared for transplantation. Only parts of the diaphragm around the suprahepatic vena cava and the celiac trunk have still to be prepared. Depending on the kind of arterial reconstruction, either a small patch from the aorta for the celiac trunk or a long conduit from the thoracic aorta was prepared. In this case all intrathoracically branching segmental arteries have to be ligated and the distal opening of the aorta has to be sutured. This should be done in a conical manner (Fig. 1). Until transplantation the liver is stored in cold perfusion solution.

5.2 OPERATION OF THE RECIPIENT ANIMAL

The operation of the recipient animal has to be performed without using a veno-venous bypass. The operation can be distributed into four phases:

I. Hepatectomy

After opening the abdomen through a median incision the liver is freed of adhesions, the ligamentum falciforme, the ligamentum triangularis sinistrum and the small net are transsected. The hepatoduodenal ligament is dissected close to the hilus: the hepatic arteries and the common bile duct are transsected very close to the liver. The portal vein is dissected from the liver to the pancreas. Then the infrahepatic vena cava is dissected, the branching veins to the suprarenal gland are separated and the infrahepatic vena cava is looped close to the branches of the renal veins. The liver is dissected from the retroperitoneum and the diaphragm. After clamping of the portal vein and the infrahepatic and suprahepatic vena cava, all vessels are transsected very close to the liver.

II. Anhepatic phase

The first step in this operative phase is to look for bleeding and to achieve complete hemostasis of the liver bed. The retroperitoneum which had to be opened in the area of the right suprarenal gland and the diaphragm dorsal of the liver is carefully sutured.

Then the anastomoses are performed. First the suprahepatic vena cava is sutured using 5/0-Prolene, then the infrahepatic vena cava is sutured by 6/0-Prolene. In some monkeys the celiac trunk along with a small aortic patch was anastomosed directly onto the recipient aorta proximal to the branching of the recipient's own celiac trunk. For this anastomosis 6/0-Prolene was used. In other monkeys arterial reconstruction was performed by an aortic conduit. In cases requiring the second procedure, anastomosing was always performed after the reperfusion. After shortening the portal vein this vessel is anastomosed using 6/0-Ethilon.

III. Reperfusion phase

After portal vein anastomosis has been completed the graft is reperfused at once. No loss of blood or fluid should be accepted; even the amount of the perfusion solution that has remained within the graft during cold storage has to flow into the systemic circulation.

IV. Postreperfusion phase

In this phase, reconstruction of the artery (if not already done) and the bile duct is performed. The aortic conduit is anastomosed onto the infrarenal part of the abdominal aorta. The right flexure of the colon is mobilized in order to avoid any tension and the anastomosis is performed using 6/0-Prolene. The bile ducts are reconstructed by using the side-to-side choledocho-choledochostomy technique. After final control of hemostasis the abdominal wall is closed.

The recipient operations were performed in about 3-1/2 hours due to the high grade of standardization. Cold ischemic time ranged between 3-1/2 to 5 hours. The anhepatic phase was 45-60 minutes and the time for the anastomoses (starting with the anastomosis of the suprahepatic vena cava until reperfusion) ranged from 35-55 minutes.

6. POSTOPERATIVE MANAGEMENT OF THE ANIMALS AND DOCUMENTATION OF THE FURTHER COURSE

Immediately after operation the animals had free access to water and they began enteral nutrition in the first few postoperative days. The general condition of the animals was monitored and documented daily especially concerning food volume, defecation, vitality, icterus etc. Whenever blood samples were taken the temperature was measured. In some animals infections or diarrhea occurred in the later course; however, these were easily treated with antibiotics in all cases.

7. BLOOD SAMPLING, LIVER BIOPSIES AND POSTMORTEM EXAMINATION

Blood was taken postoperatively just prior to the removal of the cannulas and on postoperative days 3, 7, 14, 21 and weekly in the first few months thereafter. To enable blood sampling the animals underwent brief anesthesia. The red and white blood cell count, the coagulation, bilirubin, transaminases, cholestasis-indicating enzymes and renal function parameters as well as the cyclosporin level were determined.

Liver biopsies were taken under brief anesthesia. For most animals liver biopsies are available from postoperative days 7, 14 and 21. Thereafter liver biopsies were taken at various intervals. Sometimes the biopsy material was not sufficient for adequate histological assessment, and in some animals biopsy was not performed at all regular postoperative intervals because of the risk.

Histological specimens were fixed in 10% formalin and routinely stained with hematoxylin-eosin. Each specimen was considered without knowledge of the clinical situation of the monkey. Besides the detailed description of the histological findings the so-called Hannover Classification was applied to assess the severity of acute rejection. This classification was developed in humans (see also methods of the clinical study, page 16) and distinguishes five grades of severity. (See also Table 8.) Animal specimens were re-trospectively classified. This enabled comparison within and between animal groups as well as comparison with the findings derived from the patients in the clinical part of this study.

In case of death a careful postmortem examination of the animal was performed. The liver was examined level by level, and each level was histologically classified separately. When this classification varied between the different levels this was documented and the most severe grade was taken into account for further consideration. All animals were observed for surgical complications.

RESULTS

1. SPONTANEOUS COURSE WITHOUT BASIC IMMUNOSUPPRESSION

1.1 SURVIVAL

Twenty-four animals received no immunosuppression at all after liver transplantation, neither as basic immunosuppression nor as rejection treatment. The longest survival was 116 days, the shortest one 4 days (Fig. 2). Eleven animals died within the first 9 days (median: day 6), the other animals survived 22-116 days (median: day 40).

1.2 CLINICAL FINDINGS IN THE EARLY POSTOPERATIVE PERIOD

The general condition of the monkeys became normal very quickly after successful transplantation. They started eating on the first postoperative day and their behavior became normal on days 2-3. Depending on the survival time a deterioration of the general condition occurred, worsening more or less quickly until the animal died. In 21 animals sufficient blood chemistry data of the early postoperative period are available. None of the 21 animals had absolutely normal values of bilirubin, transaminases and cholestasis-indicating enzymes. In some animals all of these parameters were strongly pathological; in other animals various grades of changes

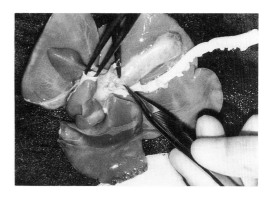

Fig. 1. Perfused and completely prepared donor liver. Artery with aortic conduit sutured in conical manner. Vena portae and vena cava marked with forceps. Biopsy area sutured.

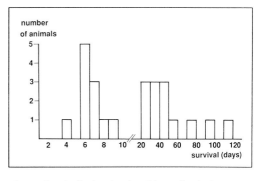

Fig. 2. Survival of animals without basic immunosuppression.

Table 1. Early postoperative histological findings of rejection in animals without immunosuppression (according to Hannover Classification)

Severity grade	A_0	A_{0-1}	A_1	A_2	A_{2-3}	A_3
Frequency	0	5	5	0	3	6

could be observed. In some animals transaminases increased, in other animals bilirubin and cholestasis-indicating enzymes were especially elevated. In most cases elevated levels of these indicators persisted. Sometimes a temporary decrease was observed; however, complete normalization of the values was never achieved, not even late in the postoperative course.

1.3 Histological findings in the early postoperative period

In 19 of 24 animals sufficient histological material for a complete evaluation could be obtained postoperatively. All animals showed more or less intense signs of rejection at the end of the first postoperative week (Table 1). In 10 animals only a slight deterioration was seen which was considered A_{0-1} or A_1 according to the Hannover Classification. In the other nine animals signs of severe acute rejection were observed and the corresponding grade of severity was A_{2-3} or A_3.

In no case was spontaneous remission of the rejection observed. Even in the animals with initially slight findings, further deterioration was observed. Some of these cases developed severe acute rejection (A_3); some developed chronic rejection in the long-term.

Strong vascular reactions (Fig. 3) and endothelitis (Fig. 4 a,b) was observed in the early postoperative period. To some extent, these changes dominated the histological picture.

Cholestasis was observed only in two animals and was presumably due to mechanical problems. In one of these two animals purulent cholangitis ensued.

In many animals a striking variety of findings was observed at the same time. On postmortem examination, strongly rejected grafts showed the severity grade A_3. However, in some strongly rejected livers also different grades of severity were observed in different areas of the whole organ. In general, this discrepancy did not exceed more than one severity grade of the Hannover Classification. Nevertheless, in two animals areas of only slight rejection with a corresponding low grade of severity (A_1) were observed in livers that revealed a strong acute rejection (A_3) in all other parts (Fig. 5a,b).

1.4 Clinical and histological features of rejection and survival

Complete clinical and histological data could be obtained from 19 animals. Depending on the severity of rejection these animals had markedly different survival times (Fig. 6).

All animals with clinical findings of acute rejection and a high histological grade of rejection (A_{2-3} or A_3) in the initial biopsy in the early postoperative period died by postoperative day 9.

In contrast, all animals demonstrating only a slight histological grade of rejection in the initial biopsy (A_{0-1} or A_1) survived this period and died later (day 22-95, median: day 34). An example is given in Figure 7. After a temporary clinical improvement on day 14 the course deteriorated and the high histological grade of severity persisted throughout the entire postoperative period. The animal, in marked rejection, died on postoperative day 22.

1.5 RhLA-COMPATIBILITY AND SURVIVAL

Complete RhLA-typing including determination of the DR-locus was available for all donor recipient pairs. The relationship between RhLA-compatibility and survival is depicted in Table 2. Differences in survival in relation to the compatibility in the A- or B-locus could not be detected. In the DR-locus most of the animals showed no compatibility. Animals with one or two compatibilities varied in their survival from 4 days up to 95 days.

An influence of RhLA-compatibility on survival could not be demonstrated.

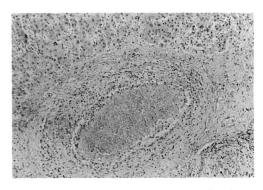

Fig. 3. Florid arteritis in interlobar area. This shows a branch of the hepatic artery with mononuclear, partly mixed infiltrates in the outer part. Animal on postoperative day 21 without immunosuppression (hematoxilin-eosine, x 270).

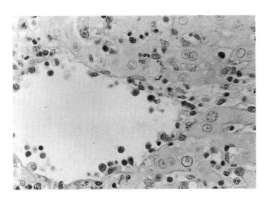

Fig. 4a: Slight endothelitis of central vein with early undermining of endothelium with inflammatory cells. Slight acute rejection grade A_1 on postoperative day 7 without immunosuppression (hematoxylin-eosin, x 400).

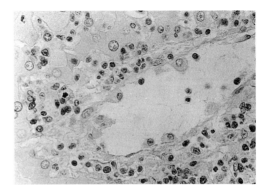

Fig. 4b: Extensive endothelitis with marked swelling of endothelia and mixed infiltrates and also with retrograde changes on central hepatocytes. Moderate acute rejection grade A_2 on postoperative day 14 without immunosuppression (hematoxylin-eosin, x 400).

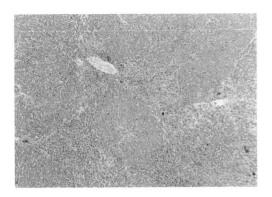

Fig. 5a: Various grades of severity of acute rejection in one area of the liver parenchyma (heterogeneity A_2 up to A_3). Postmortem material, postoperative day 7 without immunosuppression (hematoxylin-eosin, yellow filter, x 40).

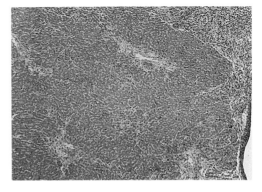

Fig. 5b: Various grades of severity of acute rejection in one area of liver parenchyma (heterogeneity A_1 up to A_3). Postmortem material, postoperative day 6 without immunosuppression (hematoxylin-eosin, blue filter, x 40).

1.6 RhLA-COMPATIBILITY AND THE CLINICAL AND HISTOLOGICAL FEATURES OF REJECTION

Statistical relationships between RhLA-compatibility and the above mentioned different features of clinical signs could not be detected. In some animals without any compatibility in the DR-locus a marked increase of bilirubin and cholestasis-indicating enzymes in conjunction with only slight deterioration of the transaminases could be observed when rejection occurred. An example is given in Figure 8.

An influence of RhLA-compatibility on histological features could not be detected.

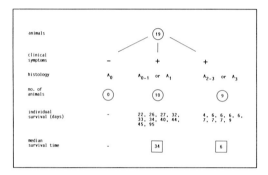

Fig. 6. Features of rejection and survival in animals without basic immunosuppression.

Table 2. RhLA-compatibility and survival without immunosuppression (spontaneous course)

| RhLA-compatibility | | Survival |
locus	number	(days)
A or B	0	6, 6, 7, 26, 32, 33, 40, 44, 116
DR	0	
A or B	1-2	6, 6, 9, 22, 45, 55, 79
DR	0	
A or B	0	7, 27
DR	1	
A or B	1-2	6, 8, 34, 95
DR	1	
A or B	0	4
DR	2	
A or B	1	7
DR	2	

2. COURSE WITH BASIC IMMUNOSUPPRESSION

2.1 SURVIVAL

Ten of 17 animals receiving basic immunosuppression after liver transplantation but no additional treatment in case of rejection survived and died only after cessation of immunosuppression (see also page 13), between days 61 and day 579 postoperatively. Two animals suffered from severe acute rejection and died on postoperative days 17 and 23 respectively. Five animals had a complicated course. This was mainly due to nonimmunological factors, partly in combi-

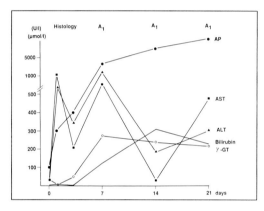

Fig. 7. Example of an animal without basic immunosuppression: acute rejection on postoperative day 7. Temporary clinical recovery, but persistence of the histological findings. Progression of rejection and death on postoperative day 22. Especially remarkable is the histological severity grade A_1 in the biopsy on the penultimate day before death.

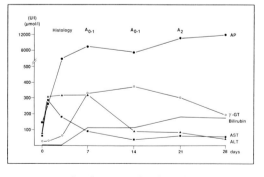

Fig. 8. Example of an animal without basic immunosuppression: acute rejection on postoperative day 7 with progression, increase in bilirubin and cholestasis dominating.

nation with immunological deterioration. These animals died on postoperative days 22, 24, 30, 30 and 55.

2.2 CLINICAL FINDINGS IN THE EARLY POSTOPERATIVE PERIOD

The normalization of the general condition of the monkeys was similar to that of the animals without basic immunosuppression. Except in animals with complicated courses or with early severe rejection, deterioration of the general condition ensued only after cessation of basic immunosuppression and was much slower than in those monkeys that did not receive basic immunosuppression and underwent rejection.

Biochemical data in the early postoperative period are available for all animals. Most show an increase either in all parameters such as transaminases, bilirubin or cholestasis-indicating enzymes or at least in some of these parameters. Some animals had normal or nearly normal values of some parameters. The further course of some of these animals is characterized by a slow increase in some parameters continuing despite permanent basic immunosuppression.

2.3 HISTOLOGICAL FINDINGS IN THE EARLY POSTOPERATIVE PERIOD

Complete biopsy specimens sufficient for a detailed examination were available for eight animals under basic immunosuppression in the early postoperative period. All of these animals had histological signs of rejection in the early postoperative phase, but none demonstrated a grade of severity higher than A_1, which means that in all cases only slight histological signs of rejection were detectable (Table 3).

In two animals the further course was characterized by a progression of the findings up to grade A_3 and early death. In the other animals the course was characterized by a decrease of the severity grade to A_0 or by persistence of the severity grade leading to the development of chronic rejection. The further course was decisively determined by the cessation of basic immunosuppression (see paragraph 3).

Vascular changes such as endothelitis in conjunction with acute rejection were detectable, however, not especially severe.

In contrast, bile duct changes were very marked especially after 4-6 postoperative weeks.

2.4 CLINICAL AND HISTOLOGICAL FEATURES OF REJECTION AND SURVIVAL

The postoperative course and survival were considerably different depending on the clinical and histological features of rejection findings in the early postoperative phase (Fig. 9). Histologically, all animals showed a slight rejection (A_{0-1} or A_1) at the end of the first

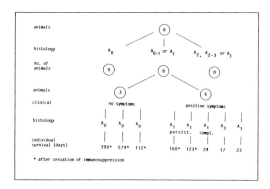

Fig. 9. *Features of rejection and survival in animals with basic immunosuppression.*

Table 3. Early postoperative histological findings of rejection in animals with basic immunosuppression (according to Hannover Classification)

Severity grade	A_0	A_{0-1}	A_1	A_2	A_{2-3}	A_3
Frequency	0	4	4	0	0	0

Table 4. RhLA-compatibility and survival with basic immunosuppression

RhLA-compatibility		Survival
Locus	number	(days)
A or B	0	23, 24[k], 30[k]
DR	0	
A or B	1-2·	30[k], 55[k], 61*, 161*, 112*, 160*, 399*, 579*·
DR	0	
A or B	0	156*
DR		
A or B	1-2	17, 22[k], 123*, 189*, 509*
DR	1	
A or B	0	·
DR	2	
A or B	1	·
DR	2	

* after cessation of immunosuppression
[k] complicated postoperative course
· 1 animal with 3 compatibilities

postoperative week. Three animals demonstrated no clinical symptoms of rejection. In these three animals the histological findings reversed spontaneously and all three survived long-term and died only after cessation of immunosuppression.

Five animals demonstrated both histological and clinical signs of rejection. The histological grade of severity was slight (A_{0-1} or A_1). None of these animals had spontaneous remission to normal, neither histologically nor clinically. In two animals a rapid progression to grade A_3 portended death of the animals on days 17 and 23, respectively. One animal died after a complicated course on postoperative day 24; in two animals findings of persistent rejection of more or less intensity were seen. Both survived long-term and died only after cessation of immunosuppression on day 123 and 160, respectively.

2.5 RhLA-compatibility and survival

Complete RhLA-typing including the DR-locus was available for all donor-recipient pairs. The relationship between RhLA-compatibility and survival is depicted in Table 4. Most of the animals revealed one or more compatibilities in the A- or B-locus; only

four animals revealed a complete mismatch. The different survival times are homogeneously distributed in all groups of different compatibility. Eleven animals revealed no compatibility, six revealed one and no animal a complete compatibility in the DR-locus. The various survival times are homogeneously distributed in this group as well.

An influence of RhLA-compatibility on survival was not demonstrated by the present material for class I nor for class II antigens.

2.6 RhLA-compatibility and the clinical and histological features of rejection

At the end of the first postoperative week 10 animals revealed clinical symptoms corresponding to acute rejection. The symptoms differed in various parameters. A relationship to RhLA-compatibility in the A- or B-locus could not be detected in contrast to the compatibility in the DR-locus (Table 5). Animals with one DR-compatibility showed complete symptomatology with an increase in transaminases, bilirubin and cholestasis-indicating enzymes. In contrast, animals with a complete mismatch in the DR-locus showed a symptomatology with an increase in bilirubin and cholestasis-indicating enzymes whereas the transaminases remained nearly normal in most cases. A relationship between the histological feature and RhLA-compatibility could not be observed.

3. COURSE AFTER CESSATION OF BASIC IMMUNOSUPPRESSION

In 10 animals basic immunosuppression was stopped after an uncomplicated course. They died between days 33 and 481. None of these animals developed permanent tolerance

(Table 6). In eight animals the immunosuppression was stopped on postoperative day 28. In three of these animals acute rejection occurred within a very short time thereafter and could be successfully treated by monoclonal antibodies. However, a second period of acute rejection followed very quickly. One of these animals died on day 61; in the other two animals a second treatment with monoclonal antibodies was successful. Both animals survived long-term, until they died of chronic rejection on days 181 and 509 respec-

Table 5. *Relationship between DR-compatibility and increase of clinical parameters typical of acute rejection in several animals depicted separately*

DR-compatibility	Increase of		
	AST, ALT	Bilirubin	γ-GT
1	+	+	+
1	+	+	+
1	+	+	+
1	*	+	+
0	–	+	+
0	–	+	+
0	–	+	+
0	–	+	+
0	+	+	+
0	*	+	+

* no data available

Table 6. *Course and survival after cessation of immunosuppression*

Postoperative day of cessation	Rejection treatment		Survival total (days)	Survival after cessation (days)
28	MAk*	1x	61	33
28	MAk*	2x	189	161
28	MAk*	2x	509	481
28	–		112	84
28	–		123	95
28	–		156	128
28	–		160	132
28	–		161	133
191	–		399	208
192	–		579	387

*MAk = treatment course with the monoclonal antibody FN 18

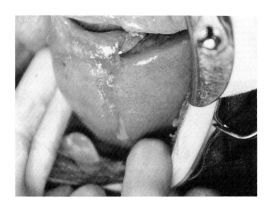

Fig. 10. Liver just after reperfusion reveals rapidly developing marbled surface and paleness.

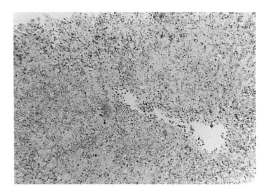

Fig. 11a. Extensive fresh hemorrhagic necrosis, namely the early stage of red hepatodystrophia in hyperacute rejection, postmortem material 3 hours after operation (hematoxylin-eosin, x 40).

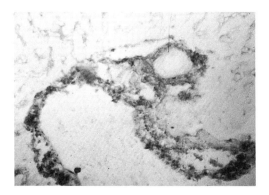

Fig. 11b. Intense immunoglobulin deposits (IgM, IgG) in vessel walls of the portal tract in hyperacute rejection; postmortem material 3 hours after operation (polyclonal antibody staining against monkey immunoglobulin—IgM, IgG, indirect immuno-peroxidase reaction, x 340).

tively. The other five animals survived without rejection therapy between days 84 and 133 until they died between days 112 and 161. In two animals basic immunosuppression was stopped on days 191 and 192. They survived without rejection treatment for a long time (208 and 387 days) and died on days 399 and 579 respectively.

4. DONOR-SPECIFIC PRESENSITIZATION

After donor specific presensitization four of six animals died within a few hours after reperfusion or on the first postoperative day. Two animals survived for 7 and 22 days respectively (Table 7).

All animals including the four surviving only a few hours after reperfusion showed good and homogeneous reperfusion. In some of the animals with very short survival macroscopic changes were already observed intraoperatively. The surface of the liver suddenly became marbled and discolored (Fig. 10). Initially the operative field was dry without any bleeding, but after a while diffuse, nonsurgical bleeding started. In one monkey a biopsy taken 30 minutes after reperfusion showed histologically, red hepatodystrophy. Histological assessment of the whole liver performed later showed degenerative or even necrotic changes of nearly all hepatocytes combined with a hemorrhagic component. One animal showed signs of a shock liver with centroacinar necrosis. In all the findings revealed focal changes with extensive hemorrhagic necrosis (Fig. 11a). The immunohistochemical staining revealed massive deposits of immunoglobulins (Fig. 11b).

Table 7. Donor-specific presensitization and survival

Donor specific presensitization		Cross-match at time of transplantation	Intraop. blood transfusion	Survival in days
blood	skin			
+	+	+	–	0
+	+	+	–	0
+	+	+	–	0
+	+	+	+	1
+	+	+	+	7
+	+	+	+	22

The two animals surviving for a longer period (days) demonstrated a different course. One animal died on postoperative day 7 with histologically extensive hemorrhagic necrosis. The other animal survived until day 22. Histology revealed severe acute rejection. These two animals as well as the animal surviving for one day received fresh blood during liver transplantation from third animals. This was not due to bleeding but to a routine procedure according to the transplantation protocol. In contrast the three animals dying a few hours after reperfusion did not receive any blood during the liver transplantation. In all three animals the operation was technically and anesthesiologically satisfactory and none of the animals would have required blood transfusions due to the operative procedures (Table 7).

Early Postoperative Rejection After Liver Transplantation

METHODS

1. PERI- AND INTRAOPERATIVE MANAGEMENT AND MONITORING

Within 19 months 98 orthotopic liver transplantations were performed in 81 adult patients consecutively in the Klinik für Abdominal- und Transplantationschirurgie, Medizinische Hochschule Hannover. The indications were an end-stage cirrhosis in 31 patients, various benign disorders other than cirrhosis in 21 patients, a malignant tumor in 17 patients and a malignant tumor in a cirrhotic liver in 12 patients.

The donor organs were evaluated and removed according to our standard procedure for multiorgan harvesting (Gubernatis 1988c, 1989e, f). Eurocollins solution was used as perfusion solution in all cases. Extracorporeal porto-femoro-axillary veno-venous bypass was used in all transplantations. Reconstruction of the bile ducts was done as a side-to-side anastomosis between the donor and the recipient common bile duct whenever possible (Neuhaus 1982). In 15 patients this kind of anastomosis was either technically not feasible or contraindicated due to the malignant primary disease. In these cases a biliodigestive anastomosis was performed using a Roux-en-Y-loop.

Postoperatively the patients were monitored intensively and continuously. Besides the general parameters such as circulation, temperature etc., hematological parameters, coagulation factors, bilirubin, transaminases and cholestasis-indicating enzymes as well as the volume of T-tube bile were assessed at least once per day. If necessary these assessments were performed several times daily. Liver biopsies were taken in the donor, in the recipient prior to and just after reperfusion and on postoperative days 7,14,21 and 28 and, in addition, whenever there was a suspicion of rejection or other deterioration that might be detectable by histological examination. Basic immunosuppression consisted of cyclosporin A and prednisolone in low dosages. Prednisolone was tapered in the postoperative course. Cyclosporin A was administered intravenously in the beginning of the postoperative period and then switched to oral administration after a stable metabolic phase with oral nutrition had been achieved. Dosages were adjusted to blood levels aiming at a therapeutic window of 500-700 ng/ml in the polyspecific RIA of the whole blood. In case of inadequate graft function or in complicated situations involving the recipient, basic immunosuppression was modified. Then triple or quadruple drug therapy was instituted partly using poly- or monospecific antibodies for 7 up to 10 days. After discharge from the hospital all patients were evaluated every two to four weeks and more frequently in case of special problems . All patients in this study were followed until death or at least for six months.

Ten patients who died early postoperatively were excluded from this study. In three patients the graft never functioned and the patients died before a second graft became available. In two patients intraoperative blood loss led to a nonfunctioning donor organ. One case was attributed to a complex operative procedure in the recipient due to multiple previous operations, and the other case led to intraoperative death. In two patients vascular thrombosis occurred and in three patients fulminant infections caused death in the first few postoperative days.

All patients except one (see "Results:

hyperacute rejection," page 27) were transplanted ABO-blood group identical, i.e., compatible, and the direct lymphocytotoxic test (cross-match) was negative (as far as available) except in four patients.

In 48 of 71 patients complete HLA-typing of the donor and the recipient including a reliable DR-assessment was available.

Graft damage after reperfusion was assessed by the early postoperative values of the transaminases and classified by using the peak levels within the first three postoperative days. The median peak levels of all patients were calculated to AST 543 U/l and ALT 473 U/l. Severe graft damage was assumed whenever one or both peak levels increased to more than 1000 U/l within the first three postoperative days.

2. FINDINGS AND DEFINITION OF ACUTE REJECTION

For the diagnosis of acute rejection three criteria were used:

1. The histological findings were classified according to the Hannover Classification of acute rejection distinguishing five grades of severity (Table 8). (See also Chapter 3.)

Table 8. Histopathological classification of liver allograft rejection—overview of the Hannover Classification

severity grade	A – 0	A – 0 – 1	A – 1	A – 2	A – 3
general characteristic	no evidence of rejection	consistent with rejection, but non–diagnostic	mild acute rejection	moderate acute rejection	severe acute rejection
infiltrates characteristic	no	slight mixed	slight mononuclear predom. lymphocytic partially mixed	more pronounced mixed predom. mononuclear	marked mixed predom. mononuclear
location		portal	portal and less parenchymal	portal and less parenchymal	portal and parenchymal
parenchyma retrogressive changes (in % hep.)	no	no	degenerative changes up to necrosis less than 10%	degenerative changes focal non–bridging necrosis 10% – 30%	pronounced degen. changes partly bridging necrosis more than 30%
endothelialitis location	no	no	+ portal or/and central	+ portal and central	+ portal and central
bile duct damage	no	less than 50%	more than 50%	more than 50%	more than 50%

in % hep. = in % of all hepatocytes
predom. = predominated
degen. = degenerated

Besides this classification, the findings of cholangitis were stated according to general histopathological criteria (Wight, 1983a). In no case was a purulent cholangitis treatable by antibiotics in our observations.

2. Besides a deterioration of the general condition of the patient, the clinical symptoms of an acute rejection were considered an increase in transaminases, glutamate dehydrogenase (GLDH), bilirubin and cholestasis-indicating enzymes and the occurrence of fever.

3. The decision regarding the necessity of rejection treatment was based on histological findings as well as on a thorough consideration of the whole clinical situation. In principle, the treatment started with daily bolus injections of 500 mg methylprednisolone for one up to three days (most frequent). In some cases this therapy was continued for five days or poly- or monoclonal antibodies were administered additionally. According to the definition of the diagnosis "acute rejection" the complete triad of histological findings, clinical symptoms and rejection therapy applied was required.

3. HISTOPATHOLOGICAL CLASSIFICATION OF LIVER ALLOGRAFT REJECTION—THE "HANNOVER-CLASSIFICATION"

The so-called Hannover Classification of liver allograft rejection is the result of our own observations and findings and the results of other studies especially Snover's (Snover 1984, 1986, 1987, see also Snover 1990). The Hannover Classification distinguishes between the various grades of severity in both acute and chronic rejection. In order to make this chapter on the Hannover Classification system more comprehensive, both types will be described in detail and histopathological examples of each level of severity will be given.

3.1 The "Hannover Classification" of Acute Rejection

Acute rejection is characterized by Snover's criteria:
1. Portal infiltrates
2. Changes of the interlobular bile ducts
3. Venous endothelitis

4. The spectrum of retrograde to necrotic changes of the liver parenchyma.

The classification distinguishes five grades of severity as follows (A as symbol for acute rejection; index 0 up to 3 as symbol for the grading):

A_0:   no sign of acute rejection
A_{0-1}: consistent with rejection but non-diagnostic
A_1:   slight acute rejection
A_2:   moderate acute rejection
A_3:   severe acute rejection.

The portal infiltrates of acute rejection in the liver parenchyma are mixed cellular infiltrates in general, partly in conjunction with single plasma cells. These infiltrates are not specific as such; the presence of infiltrates therefore does not inevitably indicate rejection. Changes in bile ducts, however, are pathognomonic for the diagnosis of an acute rejection. Venous endothelitis is also a nearly specific sign of acute rejection. The spectrum of retrograde to necrotic changes of the hepatocytes is characteristic of the various grades of severity of rejection. Nearly all types of retrograde to necrotic hepatocyte changes can occur in conjunction with acute rejection. Cholestasis is a frequent concomitant phenomenon of rejection. Our studies, however, showed that this is not an absolutely diagnostic and specific sign.

Basic elements for the histopathological diagnosis are depicted in Figure 12.

Histopathological criteria of the different grades of severity are as follows:

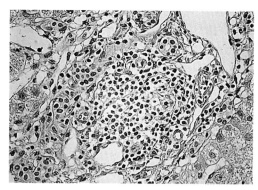

Fig. 12a. *Slight mixed portal infiltrate and mild bile duct damage (grade 1) without endothelitis.*

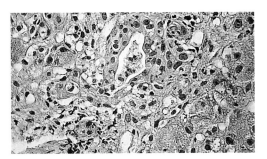

Fig. 12b. Moderate bile duct damage (grade 2) with the pleomorphism of the bile duct epithelial cells and with still intact wall of the bile duct.

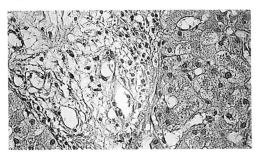

Fig. 12c. Severe bile duct damage (grade 3) with disruption of the ductular walls and with remnants of bile duct epithelial cells (resulting in so-called "vanishing bile duct syndrome").

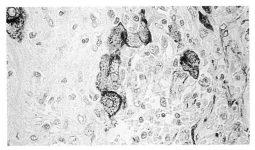

Fig. 12d. Remnants of the bile duct epithelial cell stained immunohistochemically with antibody against cytokeratin (the same case as in Fig. 12c).

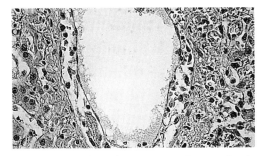

Fig. 12e. Endothelitis with retrogressive changes of endothelial cells with accumulation of lymphocytes beneath the endothelium and with marked elevation of the endothelium from its underlying basement membrane.

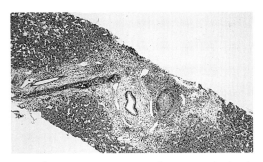

Fig. 12f. Rare event accompanying acute rejection in the portal area: partly occlusive arteritis in portal tract in biopsy, seventh day after liver transplantation.

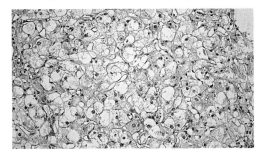

Fig. 12g. Example of retrogressive changes of hepatic parenchyma: ballooning.

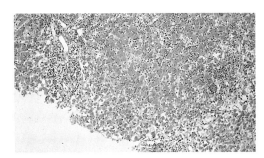

Fig. 12h. Example of retrogressive changes of hepatic parenchyma: bridging up to confluent necroses of hepatic parenchyma.

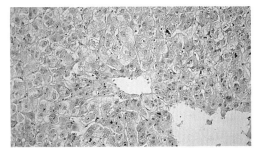

Fig. 12i. Cholestasis of moderate grade accompanied by nondiagnostic phenomenon of acute rejection.

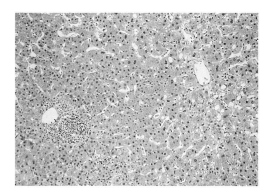

Fig. 13. Acute rejection: grade 0-1—consistent with rejection but nondiagnostic; no endothelitis.

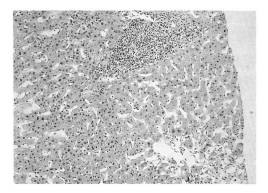

Fig. 14. Mild acute rejection: grade 1—with retrogressive changes of hepatic parenchyma involving up to 10% in biopsy material.

A_0:   no sign of acute rejection

A_{0-1}: consistent with acute rejection, but nondiagnostic (Fig. 13):

Slight mixed infiltrates, changes of bile ducts, no venous endothelitis.

A_1:   slight rejection (Fig. 14):

Slight mononuclear, predominantly lymphocytic, partly mixed cellular infiltrates in the portal tracts, venous endothelitis in portal tracts, predominantly both central and portal, changes of bile ducts, changes of the liver parenchyma—even necrosis, partly with infiltrates, involving up to 10% of all hepatocytes.

A_2:   moderate acute rejection (Fig. 15):

More pronounced intensity and density of infiltrates in portal tracts with degenerative changes of the liver parenchyma and focal, nonbridging necrosis of the liver parenchyma with mixed, predominantly mononuclear infiltrates, 10-30% of the whole liver parenchyma involved; portal and central venous endothelitis; changes of bile ducts.

A_3:   severe acute rejection (Fig. 16):

Marked inflammatory, predominantly mononuclear infiltrates in portal tracts and in the liver parenchyma with marked degenerative changes of the liver parenchyma with necrosis (more than 30% of all hepatocytes), the necroses are frequently bridging; venous endothelitis in

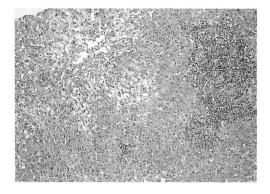

Fig. 15. Moderate acute rejection: grade 2—portal and central endothelitis, bile-duct damage G1-G2, portal infiltrates with retrogressive changes of hepatic parenchyma involving approximately 20% (10-30%).

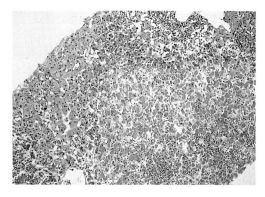

Fig. 16. Severe acute rejection: grade 3—pronounced degenerative changes and necrosis of hepatic parenchyma, involving more than 30% of all hepatocytes.

both portal and central locations and changes of bile ducts.

Histological changes of the interlobular bile ducts are as follows:

Grade 1: slight, predominantly mono-nuclear infiltrates in the epithelium with few retrograde changes of the bile ducts; bile duct wall still remaining intact.

Grade 2: pleomorphism of the bile duct epithelia with karyopyknosis or karyorrhexis, smudging of the cytoplasm, predominantly mononuclear infiltrates; however, bile duct wall still remaining intact.

Grade 3: inflammatory disruption of the bile duct wall with only a remnant of duct structures remaining up to complete disappearance of bile duct structures (vanishing bile duct syndrome).

In one individual biopsy, different grades of severity of bile duct injury may be observed simultaneously; however the most severe grade observed is decisive for the determination of the grade. In the diagnosis of A_{0-1}, the bile duct injury is present in less than 50% of all the bile ducts sampled, while the diagnosis of A_1 to A_3 implies the presence of bile duct injury in more than 50% of all bile ducts contained in the biopsy.

The resolution of the classical type of acute rejection is characterized by a decreased disappearance of the individual components of Snover's criteria. The first sign of resolution is the disappearance of the endothelitis.

3.2 The "Hannover Classification" of Chronic Rejection

The diagnosis of chronic rejection (CH) is not as self-evident as in acute rejection, the pertinent histopathological criteria being less clearly delineated. In our experience, a certain complex of changes of the portal tracts, the bile ducts, the parenchyma, and finally, the vascular system can be observed in chronic rejection. Among the changes in the portal tracts are enlargement, fibrosis (partly aggressive) and lymphocytic as well as lymphoplasmocytic infiltrates of varying intensity.

The changes observed in the portal bile ducts are similar to those occurring in acute rejection (namely grades 1-3). In addition to this, damage of hilar and trabecular bile ducts can also be observed. Advanced chronic rejection is characterized by bile duct proliferation accompanying the beginning structural alteration of the parenchyma. The parenchymal changes mainly consist in centrolobular fibrosis, which, in the progress of chronic rejection, displays the characteristics of periportal aggressive fibrosis including piecemeal necroses. The more severe the grade of chronic rejection, the higher is the degree of cholestasis (see below, I_{1-3}). Vascular changes found in chronic rejection are intimal fibrosis, subintimal foam cells up to obliterative endarteritis of the hepatic artery and clusters of foamy macrophages in sinusoidal spaces. When these changes have affected the branches of the hepatic artery, histopathologic findings corresponding to ischemic damage of the hepatic parenchyma will subsequently be observed. The terminal stage of chronic rejection is characterized by the development of cirrhosis, particularly of the micronodular type, with its typical histopathological findings.

The histopathological diagnosis of chronic rejection in percutaneous liver biopsies is rendered difficult mainly by the fact that neither larger vessels nor larger bile ducts are usually contained in the material obtained by fine-needle biopsy. However, it can be stated that the evaluation of the presence and the degree of severity of certain changes crucial for chronic rejection does allow a more or less precise diagnosis. The "Hannover Classification" distinguishes three grades of severity of chronic rejection:

CH_1: Slight chronic rejection, corresponding to chronic persistent hepatitis-like alteration

CH_2: Moderate chronic rejection, corresponding to chronic aggressive hepatitis-like alteration

CH_3: Severe chronic rejection, corresponding to cirrhosis-like alteration

Histopathological criteria of the different grades of severity are as follows:

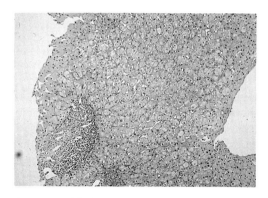

Fig. 17. Mild chronic rejection: grade 1—corresponding histopathologically to chronic persistent hepatitis-like alteration in biopsy material.

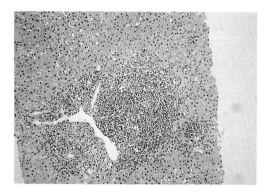

Fig. 18. Moderate chronic rejection: grade 2— corresponding histopathologically to chronic aggressive hepatitis-like alteration in biopsy material.

CH$_0$: no evidence of chronic rejection

CH$_1$: slight chronic rejection (Fig. 17):

Lobular architecture intact: portal infiltrates with predominance of lymphocytes, portal tracts clearly circumscribed, without disconnection of the portal limiting plates; changes in bile ducts and cholestasis corresponding to grade 1, I$_1$ (see below).

CH$_2$: moderate chronic rejection (Fig. 18):

Lobular architecture disturbed, but still without any signs of cirrhosis-like structural changes of parenchyma; the septa are active, the portal limiting plate shows signs of disorder; portal tracts and periportal areas with lymphocytic, partly plasmocytic infiltrates; piece-meal necroses may be present in varying extent; in the majority of the cases small clusters of foamy macrophages in sinusoidal spaces and discrete centrolobular, partly pericellular fibrosis; changes in bile ducts and cholestasis corresponding, in the majority of the cases, to grade 1-2, I$_{1-2}$ (see below);

CH$_3$: severe chronic rejection (Figs. 19-20):

Beginning structural alteration of parenchyma, to the degree of cirrhosis (pseudolobular, less frequently pseudoacinar); changes in bile ducts corresponding to grade 2-3, in cases with advanced transformation then pseudoductular proliferation; cholestasis corresponding to I$_{2-3}$ (see below).

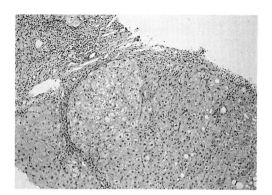

Fig. 19. Severe chronic rejection corresponding histopathologically to cirrhosis-like alteration in biopsy material.

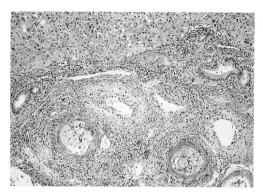

Fig. 20. Chronic rejection of vascular type with severe transplant vasculopathy in resected liver graft. It is nearly impossible to find such changes in biopsy material.

Histopathological grading of cholestasis is as follows:

For the evaluation of the type and intensity of cholestasis (symbol: I = icterus), the histopathological criteria are classified as follows:

Grade I_1: intracellular centrolobular cholestasis (Rappaport Zone 3);

Grade I_2: cholestasis as described for grade I_1, however with additional presence of canalicular cholestasis, partly also of cholestasis in v. Kupffer's cells (Rappaport Zone 3, partly involving also Zone 2); and

Grade I_3 comprising the changes occurring in grade I_1 and grade I_2, with additional ductular and finally ductal cholestasis.

Differential diagnosis of acute and chronic rejection

For the differential diagnosis of acute and chronic rejection, as well as for the diagnosis of an episode of acute rejection against the background of persistent chronic rejection, the presence of endothelitis is decisive (Kemnitz 1987). In "purely" chronic rejection, endothelitis will never occur (Kemnitz 1987, 1989a).

4. GENERAL PROCEDURE FOR EVALUATION OF ALL PATIENTS' DATA AND FINDINGS

1. In *all patients all clinical signs* potentially indicating ongoing rejection were assessed with regard to frequency, kind of expression and dynamics. This assessment was performed independently from the diagnosis of acute rejection and its definition.

2. In *all patients all histological signs* indicating an ongoing rejection were assessed concerning frequency, general circumstances and the further course. This assessment was performed independently from the diagnosis of acute rejection and its definition.

3. In *all those patients* with clinical and histological signs indicating an ongoing rejection, but *without rejection treatment* and therefore without the diagnosis of acute rejection according to its definition, the further course was assessed.

4. In *all those patients* with the diagnosis of acute rejection according to its definition and therefore *with rejection treatment,* the circumstances and the further course was assessed in detail. In order to enable standardized assessment the first day of treatment is defined as the onset of rejection. In order to evaluate the risk of acute rejection in the early and late postoperative period the first three weeks are investigated separately.

5. STATISTICAL METHODS

The present data and material represent absolute and relative frequencies. For the assessment of the frequencies and for the calculation of significance of relationships statistical methods for discrete variables are applied. The following methods are used:

5.1 CONFIDENCE LEVEL FOR THE ASSESSMENT OF FREQUENCIES ESPECIALLY IN SMALL SAMPLES

The observed relative frequency is in general different from the true value. To assess the range covering this true value with high probability the confidence level is used. For the assessment of this confidence level the number of observations in the sample survey is considered. The true value is enclosed by the confidence level with a given probability $1-\alpha$ with α as the type I error. Bunke's (Bunke 1959/60) calculated confidence levels (so-called optimal mean confidence levels) are used. The Type I error of these levels is 0.05 in the mean and always less than 0.10. The confidence levels are given in brackets after the percentage and are marked with index B.

5.2 CHI²-TEST AND CORRECTED CHI²-TEST FOR THE ASSESSMENT OF SIGNIFICANCE OF RELATIONSHIPS

For the calculation of relationships between different discrete variables the frequencies are given in the shape m x n tables respectively 2 x 2 tables (Weber 1980). It is calculated whether or not the numbers differ more than they would differ by chance on the basis of a given Type I error. The calculated test statistic is chi^2 distributed. In case the number of a sample survey is small or the frequencies are strongly unbalanced the correction by Yates (Yates 1980) is applied in addition.

RESULTS

1. CLINICAL FINDINGS IN THE EARLY POSTOPERATIVE PERIOD

Forty-four out of 71 patients revealed clinical symptoms of rejection such as the occurrence of fever, increase of bilirubin, transaminases and cholestasis-indicating enzymes within the first three postoperative weeks.

These symptoms differed in the various parameters as well as in the dynamics of their development between the patients. Some patients revealed the complete symptomatology and all parameters were changed simultaneously. Frequently only some of the parameters were abnormal. Some patients initially had only a short episode of fever of 1-3 days duration followed by an increase in bilirubin. In other patients the transaminases increased only after the bilirubin and the

cholestasis-indicating enzymes were already elevated for several days. In other patients only the transaminases increased without any change in the other parameters.

Two patients had a completely different symptomatology. They had signs of hyperacute rejection and they are therefore discussed separately.

All these findings caused by rejection varied considerably and showed no feature pathognomonic for rejection.

2. HISTOLOGICAL FINDINGS IN THE EARLY POSTOPERATIVE PERIOD

The liver biopsies from all 71 patients at the end of the first postoperative week or earlier for clinical reasons revealed histological signs of rejection in 59 patients (80%).

A detailed overview of the distribution of these histological findings is depicted in Figure 21. Courses with treated rejection are depicted on the left side, those courses with untreated rejection on the right side of the figure. In two patients histological changes indicating hyperacute rejection were demonstrated; 12 patients revealed histological grade severity A_2 in the initial biopsy and 32 patients revealed severity grade A_1. All 44 patients simultaneously had clinical signs of acute rejection and were therefore treated. Nine out of 32 patients already had previous histological signs of rejection corresponding to the severity grade A_1 without any clinical symptoms. At this time these patients as well as 13 other patients with corresponding histological findings and without any clinical symptoms were not treated. Twelve patients never demonstrated any signs of rejection in the routine biopsy within the first three postoperative weeks.

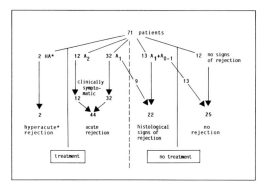

Fig. 21. Histological signs, diagnosis and treatment of early postoperative rejection.

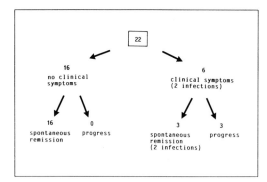

Fig. 22. Course of nontreated histological rejection.

3. CLINICAL AND HISTOLOGICAL FEATURES OF NONTREATED REJECTION AND THE FURTHER COURSE

The further course of 22 patients with findings of histological rejection but without therapeutic consequences is depicted in Fig-

Table 9. Frequency of acute rejection after liver transplantation

Patients	71	41
time of follow-up	3 weeks	6 months
acute rejection	46	25
no rejection	25	16
incidence	65%	61%

ure 22. *Sixteen patients had no clinical symptoms and all 16 had spontaneous resolution of their histological findings.* Six patients had clinical symptoms. In two patients a treatment was contraindicated due to infection; both had spontaneous remission. In three out of the four other patients the rejection symptomatology increased further.

4. FEATURES OF TREATED REJECTION IN THE EARLY POSTOPERATIVE PERIOD

In the following chapter all findings are demonstrated that were obtained from treated acute rejection according to the definition given in "Methods" (see page 16). In all these findings the complete complex of clinical symptoms, histological signs and application of treatment was given.

4.1 FREQUENCY OF EARLY POSTOPERATIVE REJECTION

Forty-one out of 71 patients had a rejection (according to the definition) in the early postoperative period. This is 65% of all transplanted patients (Table 9). Forty-one out of 71 patients were observed for six months. In this smaller group the percentage of rejection also was 61% and therefore comparable to the whole group of 71 patients.

4.2 POTENTIAL RISK FACTORS FOR EARLY POSTOPERATIVE REJECTION

The frequency of early postoperative re-

jection in relationship to the basic disease leading to the transplantation is depicted in Table 10a. Whether or not the basic disease is a malignant or benign one has no influence on the frequency of rejection (Table 10b). However, by comparing the cirrhotic status with a noncirrhotic one independent from the status of malignancy, a significantly more frequent occurrence of rejection could be calculated for the cirrhotic (Table 10c). The significance is especially high in the group of patients with malignant tumors (Table 10d).

The frequency of early postoperative rejection in relationship to the ischemic damage of the graft is depicted in Table 11.

A severely damaged graft (definition see "Methods") sustained acute rejection in 16 of 19 patients $(84\%/62.5-94.5)^B$. In contrast to these findings only 30 out of 52 patients $(57\%/45.2-73.6)^B$ with a regular, not severely damaged graft had acute rejection. The difference is significant.

The frequency of early postoperative rejection in relationship to various basic immunosuppressive regimens is depicted in Table 12 and does not reveal any differences between standardized and individualized immunosuppression.

The complex relationship between graft damage, basic immunosuppression and frequency and the histological grade of severity of rejection is depicted in Table 13. After severe graft damage it was more frequently necessary to administer immunosuppression. However, this difference is not significant (chi^2 = 1.72, α >20%). After severe graft damage higher histological grades of severity of rejection (grade A$_2$) could be seen (43%/ 20.0 - 69.2)^B in comparison to the situation after regular graft damage (20%/10.0-37.0)^B. However, this is not significant either (chi^2 = 2.62, α >10%). Independent from graft damage the histological grade of severity A$_2$ was seen in 4 of 23 patients (18%/7.2-36.8)^B receiving standardized immunosuppression. In contrast the histological grade of severity A$_2$ was seen in 8 of 21 patients (38%/19.5-59.8)^B with individualized immunosuppression (chi^2 = 2.37, α >10%). Patients with hyperacute rejection were not considered in this comparison.

*Table 10a. Overview: frequency of acute rejection in relationship
to the kind of basic disease*

Basic disease	n	Rejection	No rejection
benign	44	28	16
cirrhosis	26	18	8
other (non-cirrhotic)	18	10	8
malignant	27	18	9
tumor in cirrhosis	11	10	1
tumor without cirrhosis	16	8	8

*Table 10b. Frequency of acute rejection in
patients with benign and malignant
diseases*

	Rejection	No rejection
benign	28	16
malignant	18	9

$\chi^2 = 0.06$

*Table 10c. Frequency of acute rejection in
patients with or without cirrhosis*

	Rejection	No rejection
cirrhosis	28	9
no cirrhosis	18	16

$\chi^2 = 4.01$
$\alpha = 4.39\%$

*Table 10d. Frequency of acute rejection in
patients with or without cirrhosis
conjuncted with malignant tumor*

	Rejection	No rejection
tumor with cirrhosis	10	1
tumor without cirrhosis	8	8

$\chi^2_y = 7.02$
$\alpha_y < 1\%$

*Table 11. Frequency of acute rejection in
relationship to graft damage*

	Rejection	No rejection
severe graft damage	16	3
regular graft damage	30	22

$\chi^2 = 4.29$
$\alpha = 4.0\%$
$\chi^2_y = 3.22$
$\alpha_y = 7.8\%$

*Table 12. Frequency of acute rejection in
patients with different basic
immunosuppressive protocols*

Immunosuppression	n	Rejection	No rejection
Standardized (P, CyA)	39	25	14
Individualized	32	21	11
P CyA BMA	5	4	1
P Aza CyA	15	10	5
P Aza CyA ATG	2	1	1
P CyA ATG	2	2	–
P Aza ATG	5	2	3
P CyA P Aza	2	1	1
Hydrocortisone + low dose CyA	1	1	

P: Prednisolone
ATG: Antithymocyte globuline
CyA: Cyclosporin A
Aza: Azathioprine
BMA: Monoclonal antibody

4.3 CLINICAL AND HISTOLOGICAL FEATURES OF EARLY POSTOPERATIVE REJECTION

The onset of acute rejection episodes is depicted in Figure 23. *In most cases the onset is between postoperative day 5 and 8.* In the two patients with the onset on days 18 and 19 signs of an untreated rejection had been observed earlier. No patient was observed with initial rejection signs later than day 19.

The clinical symptomatology of rejection revealed two distinct types:

Type I is characterized by an increase in transaminases, sometimes accompanied by cholestasis.

Type II is characterized by an increase in bilirubin in combination with fever, frequently associated with severe cholestasis sometimes persisting for weeks. A clinical example for each type is given in Figures 24 and 25.

The frequency of these clinical types of rejection is depicted in Table 14. In most cases type II or a mixed type I and II was observed.

Distribution of the histological grades of severity is demonstrated in Table 15. Grade A_1 is the most frequent one followed by A_2. No patient revealed grade of severity A_3 in the first biopsy that shows signs of rejection.

The relationship between the histological grade of severity and the histological findings of cholangitis is demonstrated in Table 16. No relationship was observed between the histological grade of severity and the clinical type of rejection. However, cholangitis was only observed in conjunction with clinical type II or the combination of types I and II.

Hyperacute rejection

Two patients demonstrated features of rejection completely in the histological and clinical findings in acute rejection. These findings indicated hyperacute rejection and are therefore described separately as follows:

Case history 1

A 25-year-old man suffered from a Budd-Chiari syndrome. After conservative treatment consisting of two attempts at lysis failed and his general condition worsened, liver trans-

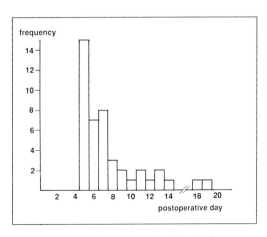

Fig. 23. Acute rejection. Depicted is the frequency of the first day at which rejection treatment was applied.

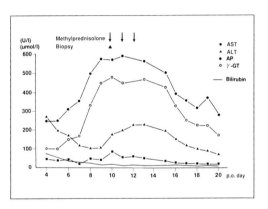

Fig. 24. Example of acute rejection of the clinical type I with predominant increase of transaminases and cholestasis-indicating enzymes.

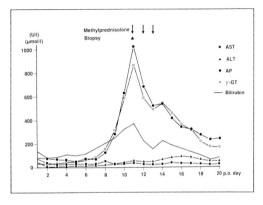

Fig. 25. Example of acute rejection of the clinical type II with a predominant increase of bilirubin and cholestasis-indicating enzymes.

plantation was undertaken. The first graft was ABO-identical and seemed to be well qualified. However, it failed completely showing signs of irreversible initial nonfunction. Urgent retransplantation became necessary and on the fourth day after the first transplantation, the patient was regrafted using an ABO-incompatible liver (donor AB, recipient A). This graft functioned during the first few postoperative days, but then deteriorated suddenly, and the histological specimens revealed signs of severe acute rejection and the need for a third transplantation was determined. The third graft was ABO-identical and transplanted five days after the second transplantation. It was an excellent graft from a 14-year-old good donor. The transplantation was uncomplicated, blood loss was low. Reperfu-

Table 13. Graft damage, basic immunosuppressive protocols, frequency and histological grade of severity in early postoperative rejection

Graft Damage	Basic Immuno-suppression	n	No rejection	Rejection	According to severity grades	According to severity grades independent from basic immunosuppression
severe graft damage	Standard	8	1	7	3 A_{0-1}/A_1 2 A_2 2 hyperacute	8 A_{0-1}/A_1 6 A_2
	Individ.	11	2	9	5 A_{0-1}/A_1 4 A_2	2 hyperacute
regular graft damage	Standard	31	13	18	16 A_1 2 A_2	24 A_{0-1}/A_2 6 A_2
	Individ.	21	9	12	8 A_{0-1}/A_1 4 A_2	

Table 14. Frequency of different clinical features in case of histologically proven and treatment-requiring acute rejection

Clinical Type	I	II	I+II	n
Frequency	9	19	15	43*

*2 patients not classified due to hyperacute rejection
 1 patient not classified because symptomatology was influenced by factors other than rejection

Table 15. Frequency of histological grades of severity in the initial biopsy in case of clinically symptomatic and treatment-requiring acute rejection

Severity	A_{0-1}	A_1	A_2	A_3	n
Frequency	4	28	12	0	44*

*2 patients not classifed due to hyperacute rejection

Table 16. Histological severity grade, histological cholangitis and clinical features of acute rejection

Histological Severity Grade	Clinical Type	Frequency Acute Rejection	Histological Cholangitis
0-1	I	1	0
	II	0	0
	I+II	3	0
1	I	6	0
	II	12	4
	I+II	9	2
2	I	2	0
	II	7	2
	I+II	3	0

sion was excellent and total oxygen consumption increased immediately. However, at the end of the operation the surface of the liver suddenly became marbled and discolored. A biopsy specimen taken at this time and examined by frozen section at once, already indicated changes of which the complete symptomatology could be seen 24 hours later, when the next biopsy specimen was taken: 20-25% of all hepatocytes were regressive to necrotic, especially in the centroacinar areas, and Snover's triad had developed. Severe intracellular and intracanalicular cholestasis was detected. Immunohistological staining revealed a T-cell: B-cell ratio of 5:4 and a marked increase of granulocytes. Deposits of IgM, IgG, IgA, C-3 complement component and fibrinogen were noted subendothelially, especially in the area of regressive and necrotic changes in hepatocytes. In these areas properdine was detectable as well (Fig. 26a and b).

Tissue typing of the AB0-identical graft revealed complete mismatches for both class I and class II antigens, but cross-match was negative.

The graft did not recover. As the condition of this young patient was still accept-able, a fourth transplantation with another AB0-identical graft was performed four days after the previous retransplantation. A reliable cross-match was not available. This graft functioned from the beginning. No signs of rejection, neither acute nor hyperacute, occurred. On day 32 after the last transplantation the patient died from infectious complications.

Case history 2
In the second patient a corresponding feature developed:

A 21-year-old woman was transplanted emergently. She was in deep coma without any reaction to pain (classification by Lücking, modified by Brunner (Brunner, 1986). The underlying pathology was cirrhosis due to Wilson's disease. The recipient's blood group was B. However, due to the emergency nature of the operation a donor organ with blood group 0 had to be accepted. The quality of the organ was considered good, the operation was unremarkable and generally uncomplicated, but due to severe portal hypertension in conjunction with coagulation disorders 12 units of blood substitutes were required. Immediate graft function was detectable. Total oxygen consumption increased markedly within a few minutes (Fig. 27), bile production was seen intraoperatively, and six hours later the patient regained consciousness. The patient's general condition improved, and immunosuppression was started with prednisolone and cyclosporin A.

On the second postoperative day liver function deteriorated suddenly: bile production and clotting factors decreased and transaminases increased. In order to exclude a vascular problem angiography was performed showing patent vessels and anastomoses but reduced intraparenchymal blood flow. Because of the undetermined nature of the problem a diagnostic laparotomy was performed. All anastomosed vessels were patent, but the liver was swollen, had a solid consistency and a discolored surface. A large biopsy was taken.

The histopathological changes revealed regressive to necrotic changes, especially centroacinar hepatocytes, and portal infiltrates.

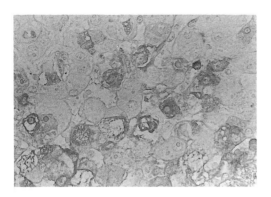

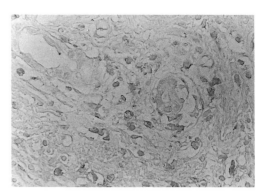

Fig. 26a. Extensive retrograde to necrotic changes of hepatocytes with strong positivity of C3 complement component in the intermediate zone. (antigen: C3 complement component, immunoalkaline phosphatase reaction, x 380).

Fig. 26b. Slight infiltrates of B-cells in a portal tract (marked by monoclonal antibodies B-cell L26 (CD21) immunoalkaline phosphatase reaction, x 300).

Fig. 27. Course of total oxygen consumption (VO$_2$) during the hepatectomy, anhepatic phase and 30 min and 90 min after reperfusion in

▲–▲ *125 patients with good primary graft function*
●–● *4 patients with irreversible initial nonfunction*
■–■ *1 patient with hyperacute rejection*

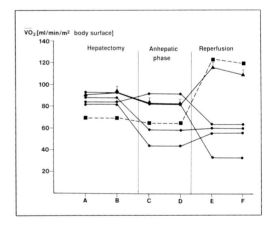

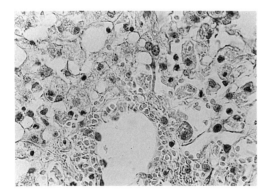

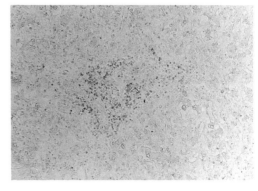

Fig. 28a. Retrograde to necrotic changes in hepatocytes surrounding a major branch of the central vein with hemorrhage and slight, early endothelitis (van Gieson-Ela, x 350).

Fig. 28b. Increase of T-cells in the infiltrates of a portal tract (marked with monoclonal antibody PAN T (CD4,8), immunoalkaline phosphatase reaction, x 45).

Table 17. Frequency of acute rejection in patients with different HLA-compatibilities

compatibility locus number	A or B 0	DR 0	A or B 1-2	DR 0	A or B 0	DR 1	A or B 1-2	DR 1
patients	13		21		7		7	
rejection	9		14		6		5	
no rejeciton	4		7		1		2	

Endothelitis, typical of acute rejection (Snover 1987) was not detectable, and bile duct changes were very minimal (Fig. 28a).

The immunohistological findings (Fig. 28b) revealed a marked increase in T-cells in portal infiltrates (T-cell: B-cell ratio 15:1). At the branches of the arteria hepatica, vena portae and vena centralis slightly subendothelial deposits of IgG, C-3 complement component, fibrinogen and—in several vessels—deposits of IgA and IgM could be detected. The areas of hepatocyte damage furthermore revealed massive deposits of IgG, IgM, IgA, C-3 complement component, properdine and fibrinogen. Furthermore IgM and IgG deposits of the membraneous type could be detected at the hepatocytes.

At this time HLA-compatibility analyzed retrospectively became known: tissue typing revealed a complete mismatch in both class I- and class II-antigens, and the cross-match was strongly positive.

Diagnosis of hyperacute rejection was established and the indication for retransplantation was made at once. Unfortunately a second graft was not available in time; the patient worsened rapidly and died on the fifth postoperative day due to complete liver failure.

Postmortem histology of the graft showed an increase of the destructive and necrotic changes in hepatocytes, an increase in portal infiltrates and focal presence of Snover's triad (Snover 1987). Cholestasis could be detected intracellularly and intracanalicularly. The immunohistological changes were the same as described above (T-cell: B-cell ratio 9:1).

4.4 HLA-COMPATIBILITY AND ACUTE REJECTION

Complete typing of donor and recipient in the HLA-A, -B and -DR-system was available for 34 patients with acute rejection early postoperatively and 14 patients without signs of rejection within the first six postoperative months (Table 17). Thirteen patients had not even a single compatibility in class I or in class II. Twenty-one patients had one or two compatibilities in the A- or B-locus, 14 patients demonstrated one compatibility in the DR-locus, one-half of the patients with and the other half without compatibility in the A- or B-locus. Complete compatibility in the DR-locus or more than two compatibilities in the A- or B-locus were never observed.

Table 18. HLA-compatibility and clinical features of acute rejeciton

HLA-compatibility locus	number	I	II	I+II
no		0	5	4
A or B DR	1-2 0	1	9	4
A or B DR	0 1	5	0	1
A or B DR	1-2 1	2	1	2

Table 19. HLA-compatibility and histological findings of acute rejection

HLA-compatibility locus	number	Severity grade* A_{0-1}	A_1	A_2	Cholangitis
no		1	5	3	2
A or B DR	1-2 0	2	8	4	5
A or B DR	0 1	1	4	1	0
A or B DR	1-2	0	2	3	0

*Hannover Classification

The frequency of acute rejection was similar in all groups of different compatibilities.

The clinical features regarding HLA-compatibility are depicted in Table 18 and reveal a close relationship to the HLA-DR-compatibility: in case of an acute rejection patients with a complete DR-mismatch showed the clinical type II or the mixed type with type II as the predominating. Patients with one DR-compatibility had mostly type I or the mixed type with type I predominating. A relationship between the clinical feature and the compatibilities in the A-or B-locus was not detectable.

The histological feature in conjunction with the HLA-compatibility is depicted in

Table 20. Treatment of acute rejection and results

Treatment	n	Reversible	Irreversible
1-3 x 500 mg methyl-prednisolone	22	20*	2
4-5 x 500 mg methyl-prednisolone	7	6	1
n x 500 mg methyl-prednisolone + antibodies	11	6**	5

* 1 patient died later due to infection
** 2 patients died later due to infection

Table 21. Treatment of acute rejection and results in relationship to basic immunosuppression

Treatment	Standardized immunosuppression reversible	irreversible	Individualized immunosuppression reversible	irreversible
1-3 x 500 mg methyl-prednisolone	11*	1	9	1
4-5 x 500 mg methyl-prednisolone	4	–	2	1
n x 500 mg methyl-prednisolone + antibodies	3*	4	3*	1

*1 patient died later due to infection
6 patients not accounted:
    2 due to arterial problems; 2 due to hyperacute rejection; 2 treatment contraindicated

Table 19. The finding of cholangitis was exclusively observed in patients completely mismatched at the DR-locus. The frequency of the various grades of severity according to the Hannover Classification was similar in all groups of various compatibilities. The patients with the best compatibility had the grade of severity A_2 more frequently than A_1. However, the numbers are small.

4.5 TREATMENT OF ACUTE REJECTION

The treatment of acute rejection is shown in Table 20. Most rejections could successfully be treated by three boluses of 500 mg methylprednisolone/day each. Even if this therapy was not totally adequate and the number of boluses had to be increased to 4-5, success could be expected in most cases. In contrast to these findings, failure of the treatment had to be expected in patients in whom the additional use of poly- or monoclonal antibodies was necessary. In these patients a

high risk $(45\%/22.5-70.0)^B$ for irreversible rejection was determined. After administration of antibodies the additional risk for lethal infection at a later time was calculated to be more likely than without antibodies. Taking these patients into account the likelihood that the steroid-resistant, antibody-requiring rejection is either irreversible or followed by infection with ensuing death is increased to 64% $(33.6-84.2)^B$. In contrast to these findings the likelihood that less severe rejections treatable by five boluses of methylprednisolone are either irreversible or followed by infection and death is only 14% $(5.6-30.3)^B$. The difference is highly significant (chi^2=9.9, α <1%/ chi^2_y=7.6, α_y < 1%).

According to the findings depicted in Table 21 the response to rejection treatment did not depend on the basic immunosuppression.

Table 22 describes the treatment and its effectiveness with regard to the different clini-

Table 22. Treatment of acute rejection and results of relationship to the clinical type of rejection

Clinical Type	Treatment	n	Reversible	Irreversible
I	1-3 x 500 mg methyl-prednisolone	6	6	-
	4-5 x 500 mg methyl-prednisolone	2	1	1
	n x 500 mg methyl-prednisolone +antibodies	1	-	1
II	1-3 x 500 mg methyl-prednisolone	9	8	1
	4-5 x 500 mg methyl-prednisolone	4	3	1
	n x 500 mg methyl-prednisolone +antibodies	4	2	2
I + II	1-3 x 500 mg methyl-prednisolone	7	6	1
	4-5 x 500 mg methyl-prednisolone	2	2	-
	n x 500 mg methyl-prednisolone +antibodies	5	4	1

cal features: type I seemed to be more easily and more effectively treatable than type II or the mixed type I and II in which antibodies had to be used more frequently. However, the difference is statistically not significant.

Most of the patients with initial histological findings of slight rejection could be treated successfully by bolus steroids in nearly all cases (Table 23). Only 17% (7.9-34.2)[B] of the patients required antibodies additionally. On the other hand patients with initial histologically moderate rejection (severity grade A_2) much more frequently required antibodies additionally (45%/22.5-70.0)[B] and were burdened with correspondingly less good results.

The effectiveness of the treatment revealed no relationship to HLA-DR-compatibility (Table 24).

4.6 RISK OF RECURRENCE AFTER REVERSIBLE REJECTION

After a successfully treated and completely reversed rejection with regard to both clinical and histological signs, a few patients suffered recurrent rejection (44%/25.7-63.69)[B]. (See

also the following paragraph "4.7 prognosis".) The clinical type of rejection remained the same in all cases (Fig. 29). As Table 25 demonstrates, a rejection of the clinical type I seemed to be followed by recurrent rejection more frequently (71%/33.1-92.7)[B] than a rejection of the clinical type II (40%/17.5-70.9)[B] or of the mixed type I and II (25%/6.4-61.2)[B]. The risk of recurrence in relationship to the histological grade of severity of the first rejection is depicted in Table 26 together with the clinical feature of rejection. This table demonstrates a homogeneous distribution of the histological and clinical features and the risk for recurrence for further rejections. As Table 27 shows the recurrence of rejection is more frequent in patients with one HLA-DR-compatibility than in patients with a complete mismatch in the DR-locus. However, this difference is statistically not significant (chi^2_y=2,5 α_y >10%). The histological grade of severity plays no role in this respect.

4.7 PROGNOSIS OF ACUTE REJECTION

Forty-six of 71 patients suffered acute rejection in the early postoperative course

Table 23. Treatment of acute rejection and results in relationship to the histological grade of severity

Histology	Treatment	n	Reversible	Irreversible
A_{0-1} or A_1	1-3 x 500 mg methyl-prednisolone	18	17*	1
	4-5 x 500 mg methyl-prednisolone	6	6	-
	n x 500 mg methyl-prednisolone +antibodies	5	3**	2
A_2	1-3 x 500 mg methyl-prednisolone	4	3	1
	4-5 x 500 mg methyl-prednisolone	2	1	1
	n x 500 mg methyl-prednisolone + antibodies	5	2	3

*1 patient died later due to infection
**2 patients died later due to infection

Table 24. Treatment of acute rejection and results in relationship to the HLA-DR-compatibility

HLA-DR compatibility	Treatment	n	Reversible	Irreversible
0	1-3 x 500 mg methyl-prednisolone	11	10	1
	4-5 x 500 mg methyl-prednisolone	4	4	-
	n x 500 mg methyl-prednisolone +antibodies	6	4	2
1	1-3 x 500 mg methyl-prednisolone	4	4	-
	4-5 x 500 mg methyl-prednisolone	2	1	1
	n x 500 mg methyl-prednisolone +antibodies	5	2	3

Table 25. Risk of recurrent rejection after successfully treated first rejection in relationship to the clinical feature of rejection (observation period 6 months)

	n	recurr. rej.
total	25	11
I	7	5
II	10	4
I+II	8	2

Table 26. Risk of recurrent rejection after successfully treated first rejection in relationship to the histological grade of severity and the clinical type of rejection (observation period 6 months)

Severity grade	Course	n	Clinical type
A_{0-1}	recurrence	1	I
	no recurr.	2	I+II, I+II
A_1	recurrence	8	I,I,I,I(chron.), II,II,II,I+II
	no recurr.	8	I,I,II,II,II,I+II,I+II,I+II
A_2	recurrence	2	II,I+II(chron.)
	no recurr.	4	II,II,II,I+II

Table 27. Risk of recurrent rejection after successfully treated first rejection in relationship to the HLA-DR-compatibility (observation period 6 months)

HLA-DR compat.	Histological severity grade	n	recurr. rej.
0	total	15	5
	A_{0-1}	2	0
	A_1	8	3
	A_2	5	2
1	total	6	5
	A_{0-1}	1	1
	A_1	4	3
	A_2	1	1

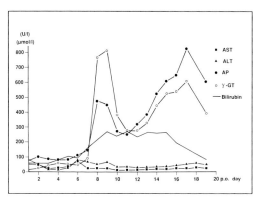

Fig. 29. Example of a recurrent rejection with the identical rejection feature type II (both episodes were treated by 3x500 mg methylprednisolone each).

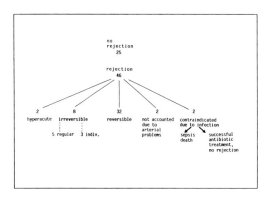

Fig. 30. Risk and prognosis of acute rejection

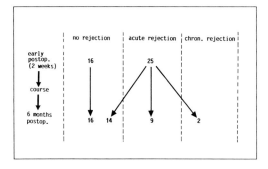

Fig. 31. Long-term risk of acute rejection for further rejection episodes (observation period six months).

(three weeks) (Fig. 30). In 10 patients rejection was irreversible—two of these patients revealed signs of hyperacute rejection. In 32 patients rejection could be successfully treated and was therefore reversible. In two patients the course of rejection was not considerable due to vascular problems. In two other patients treatment was contraindicated due to infection—one of these two patients survived this situation with antibiotic treatment.

The long-term (6-month) risk of rejection in patients with either no or successfully treated and therefore reversible acute rejection in the early postoperative course is depicted in Figure 31. All patients without rejection in the first three weeks after transplantation remained free from rejection for the further course. Fourteen of 25 patients (56%/36.4-74.3)[B] with reversible rejection remained free of rejection in the later course, whereas 9 patients (36%/19.2-55.1)[B] had recurrent acute rejection and 2 patients (8%/1.9-24.0)[B] chronic rejection during the following observation period. In summary about 70% (73%/58.2-85.0)[B] of the patients remained free from rejection in the long-term run after the early postoperative period.

EARLY POSTOPERATIVE REJECTION AFTER LIVER TRANSPLANTATION

D evelopment in medicine requires clinical observations. However, due to the paucity of opportunity for or restricted possibilities for clarification of such observations, experiments are frequently required as a supplement. The present study represents such a combination of clinical and experimental analysis. It concerns a crucial issue in liver transplantation: the appearance and relevance of early immune reactions.

The essential overall result is the proof—and the confirmation—of the relevance of early immune reactions in both the experimental model without any immunosuppression and the experimental and clinical situation with immunosuppression. The relevance but also the limits of clinical and pathohistological diagnosis of immunoreactions are shown, and it can be demonstrated that both are necessary for the correct and prompt diagnosis and treatment of rejection. Furthermore, in the field of liver transplantation as yet not known early rejection processes like hyperacute immunoreactions were observed and are analyzed.

GENERAL REMARKS

Knowledge and opinions on the relevance of immune alloreactions in experimental as well as in clinical liver transplantation have changed several times. Due to experimental findings, especially those of R. Calne and coworkers, it was thought for a long time that the liver is an immunologically privileged organ in principle: after allotransplantation of the liver animals survived without immunosuppression for a long time (Calne 1967a, 1967 b, 1969, Terblanche 1967, Pencock 1967, Riddel 1968, Starzl 1969, Garnier 1970, Gent 1971, Struck 1977). Tolerogenic properties were attributed to the liver, e.g., for the acceptance of other organs transplanted simultaneously or consecutively with the liver and genetically identical to the liver donor (Calne 1969b). This belief in the secondary importance of immunological reaction in experimental liver transplantation—in comparison to kidney transplantation— predominated in the last two decades (Calne 1983a). The reasons may be mainly due to the overriding manifestations of many other complications obscuring the immunological response or leading to early postoperative death prior to the development of the immunological response. Furthermore long-term survival in spite of immunoreactions that have taken place is obviously possible and is more easily achievable in comparison to the situation after kidney transplantation. This concerns both the spontaneous course (Starzl 1965, Binns 1967, Bockhorn 1971) and the situation under basic immunosuppression (Pichlmayr 1968).

On the other hand, even in the early years findings and opinions were present indicating that immunoreactions play a major role even in liver transplantation, e.g., in some animal models such as in the monkey (Myburgh and Smit 1975, Myburgh 1980) liver grafts were typically rejected within a very short time. More frequent and longer survival was achieved in dogs only by administering basic immunosuppression (Mikaeloff 1965, Fonkalsrud 1966, Fonkalsrud 1967, Stuart 1967). To some extent the administration of polyclonal antibodies (Starzl 1966, Huntley 1966, Mikaeloff 1967, Pichlmayr 1968, Birtch 1968) was necessary. In fact, as early as 1965 Starzl reported that rejection was the main postoperative problem in the dog model.

In spite of the recognition that immunological responses play a major role in liver transplantation many observations remain open concerning its interpretation, e.g., the "tolerogenic" effect of combined liver and kidney transplantation (Fung 1987a and b, Margreiter 1988, Eid 1990) and the obviously minor sensitivity of liver grafts to humoral reactions (Gordon 1986, Iwatsuki 1981, Calne 1979, Starzl 1974, Moor 1987). However, it is ever more apparent that cellular immunoreactions—the typical acute rejection as well as chronic rejection—are of considerable relevance for the overall results of liver transplantation. This study concerns the prompt diagnosis and treatment of the immunological response in liver transplantation, particularly with regard to the influence of histocompatibility on this response.

DIAGNOSIS OF "ACUTE REJECTION"

The diagnosis of "rejection" in the early postoperative period is complicated by two problems: 1. One must distinguish rejection from other causes of graft deterioration and 2. when one makes the diagnosis of rejection the benefits of various treatments must be weighed against their risks.

Concerning 1: Graft deterioration in the very early postoperative period can be caused by several factors such as initial nonfunction, arterial problems and infection. Rejection is only one of the possibilities and differentiation by biochemical or clinical data alone is difficult or impossible (Calne 1983b, Pichlmayr 1983, Esquivel 1985, Kirby 1987, Ascher 1988, Klintmalm 1989, Paintaud 1991). This is especially true because no findings are absolutely pathognomonic for acute rejection. On the contrary, the presentation of acute rejection is highly variable. Clinical data such as bile flow, fever, postoperative day of the onset and the course of deterioration combined with histology, bacteriology, angiography et cetra can distinguish acute rejection from other causes of graft deterioration.

Initial nonfunction of the liver graft is characterized by diminished bile production and metabolic capacity after reperfusion. If the graft damage is irreversible, death will ensue unless retransplantation is performed within a very short time. Due to the rapidity of organ failure, there is not enough time for the development of a full-blown acute cellular rejection. If graft damage is reversible without retransplantation, transaminases will decrease after the second postoperative day. The situation will become normal slowly and continuously as long as no other set-back occurs. The distinction between reversibility and irreversibility is in general very difficult (Gubernatis 1988a, Gubernatis 1988b, Gubernatis 1989a) and requires additional diagnostic tools such as total oxygen consumption or ketone-body-ratio (Bornscheuer 1988, Gubernatis 1989b, Taki 1990, Ozaki 1991, Takada 1992). If graft damage is very severe and the normalization of ischemic signs is slow, the recognition and interpretation of the clinical signs of rejection can be especially difficult. In such cases clinical signs reveal only a slowing down or a persistence in the process of normalization. In most cases the distinction between initial nonfunction and acute rejection is easily made. However, the distinction between initial nonfunction and an antibody-mediated immunological reaction like hyperacute rejection can be extremely difficult (Gubernatis 1989d). This problem is therefore described separately.

A disorder in the arterial blood supply can always occur, especially in the early postoperative period, for which there is no pathognomonic sign. On the contrary, it is extremely dependent on the time after transplantation (Tzakis 1985, Hesseling 1989 a and b). Very early in the postoperative period disorders of arterial supply cause rapid deterioration of graft function. A relatively homogeneous pattern of enzymes elevation occurs. Especially characteristic is an increase in glutamate dehydrogenase (GLDH) far in excess of increases in the transaminases. In response to this enzyme pattern, Doppler sonography or angiography was performed in each case of this study, even if the suspicion was only very slight. In this way arterial disorders could be reliably distinguished from acute rejection. Later in the postoperative period, disorders of the arterial blood supply manifest as septic complications or as chronic deterioration of graft function.

Infection in the early postoperative period usually are bacterial or fungal. Viral infections generally occur later in the postoperative course. Early infections present with marked elevations of temperature, a clinical picture compatible with sepsis and positive blood cultures. Liver function is not or only mildly compromised.

The distinction between acute rejection and cholestasis or cholangitis is much more difficult. Mechanically caused cholestasis can easily be determined by an X-ray of the T-tube (if a T-tube is in place) or by ultrasound, and purulent cholangitis can be proved by positive bacterial findings and cultures from the bile. However, nonmechanically caused cholestasis and nonpurulent cholangitis are difficult diagnostic problems. Both can occur as a hepatocellular disorder due to toxic substances or as epiphenomen in conjunction with rejection. The difficulty in distinguishing either from rejection is at least in part compounded by the fact that distinctive histological findings of rejection are at least in part based on changes in bile ducts (Adams 1987, Kemnitz 1989a). The diagnosis of isolated, primary cholestasis neither mechanically caused nor combined with rejection therefore requires repeated exclusion of rejection.

The diagnosis "acute rejection" can be established and distinguished from disorders other than these mentioned by the clinical presentation. On the other hand, if several disorders with similar clinical signs coexist with the signs of rejection, diagnosis is not possible by clinical evaluation alone, especially since the signs of rejection are variable and no pathognomonic sign or pattern of signs exists (Foster 1988, Sankary 1988, Maury 1988). Histological examination is therefore essential. Yet despite the fact that typical histological findings and patterns of findings have been developed and described for making the diagnosis of acute rejection (Wight 1983a, Snover 1984, Egging 1984, Vierling 1985, Demetris 1985, Snover 1986, Snover 1987, Adams 1987, Kemnitz 1986, Kemnitz 1987, Porter 1988, Snover 1989, Adams 1990), no pathognomonic histological sign or pattern exist for rejection (Georgii 1986, Ray 1988). There are some histological signs very characteristic for certain disorders (Wight 1983b, Georgii 1986, Kemnitz 1989c), but histology alone is not sufficient. (See also: Relevance of histological findings for the diagnosis, page 40.)

As a result, a distinction between immunological and nonimmunological causes of graft deterioration can only be made by both the clinical presentation and the histological findings.

Concerning 2: The second problem is the determination of when and how aggressively acute rejection should be treated. To solve this question the quantification of the clinical picture and histological findings are necessary.

Such a quantification does not yet exist in this field. Neither the levels of transaminases and bilirubin nor the speed at which they become elevated indicate the severity of rejection. It is believed that these laboratory findings can only be interpreted as normal or pathological, no rejection or rejection. However, in this study a distinction between various patterns of enzyme elevations could be detected. Yet the understanding of these patterns is still only descriptive in nature. The findings are not sufficient for a comprehensive quantification or classification of these patterns. Nevertheless this data could be an important new starting point of future research in this area.

The evaluation of the classical histological changes of rejection and the quantification of the grades of deterioration was performed according to the so-called Hannover Classification developed by Kemnitz. The first description was published in 1986 (Kemnitz 1986). The classification was comprehensively described above. (See also Clinical Study: Methods, page 16.) Five grades can be distinguished; besides normal findings (A_0) four grades of rejection are defined: mild (A_1), moderate (A_2) up to severe (A_3), and, in addition, a grade of transition from the still normal to mild rejection, grade (A_{0-1}), was established. In stage (A_{0-1}) all of the classic signs of rejection (Snover 1984) are still not present. However, the whole picture is consistent with rejection. The Hannover Classification is a tool for the histological quantification of rejection.

Remark: The question arises regarding the way in which immunological markers can contribute to the diagnosis of rejection, differentiating it from other causes of graft dysfunction. This field will not be considered here. Yet regarding the current status of this field, it can be said that this area holds much promise. In the future this field will become much more important, especially in conjunction with other methods such as the fine needle biopsy (see Chapter 2), bile cytology (Oldhafer 1989, Kubota 1989, Oldhafer 1990, Kubota 1990, Roberti 1992), and particularly the assessment of lymphokines, adhesion molecules etc. (Steinhoff 1990b, Behrend 1991, Hoffmann 1991).

RELEVANCE OF HISTOLOGICAL FINDINGS FOR DIAGNOSIS

In more than 80% of patients and in all animals histological signs of rejection were detectable in the early postoperative period (Fig. 9, 21). In contrast the number of rejection episodes requiring treatment in the patients was only 61% and therefore remarkably less. This probably does not mean that patients who required treatment were not treated. This can easily be seen in the animals

receiving basic immunosuppression (Fig. 9). Some of the animals did not show any signs of rejection in the consecutive biopsies (A_0), other animals showed persistent signs of acute rejection for a long time and only two animals showed a rapid progression to death within three weeks. A corresponding situation could be detected in that portion of the patient population that was not treated for rejection in spite of the presence of histological evidence of rejection (Fig. 22). Only a few of the patients progressed further while other patients had a remission and continued along an uneventful course. A prospective distinction between those experimental animals or patients requiring treatment and those for whom treatment can be withheld is not possible on the basis of the biopsy findings alone. That decision requires that the histological findings be viewed in the context of the patient's clinical presentation. All animals with histological evidence of acute rejection without any clinical symptoms underwent resolution of the histological findings in contrast to those animals with histological evidence of acute rejection and positive clinical signs of rejection. Likewise, all those patients with histological evidence of acute rejection but without any clinical symptoms of rejection had an uneventful course. The patients with histologic findings of acute rejection and a clinical picture consistent with rejection were not so homogeneous, however. Patients for whom treatment of rejection was contraindicated due to infection remitted spontaneously. Specific reasons for this could not be determined. In three of four patients whose presentation of acute rejection was apparently not considered severe enough to require treatment as graft dysfunction progressed. (Retrospectively this should be considered a wrong decision, because the symptoms were obviously present and severe enough.) Even if the absolute numbers are small, the following conclusions should be drawn regarding the relationship between the experimental and clinical findings:

A histological finding of rejection can be expected in most liver-transplanted patients in the early postoperative period. This finding alone is not an indication that treatment of acute rejection is required. *Only the combination of histological findings and a clinical picture compatible with acute rejection is an indication for immediate treatment. The failure or the delay of treatment in such a situation will lead generally to the progression of rejection.*

Therefore, regarding liver transplantation, the following very important statement can be made:

Routine biopsies for early detection of rejection after liver transplantations are not necessary. A biopsy should only be taken in case of clinical suspicion of acute rejection because histological evidence of acute rejection without supporting clinical findings is not adequate to make the diagnosis.

With regard to the histological grades of severity of acute rejection it can be stated that in the patients as well as in all animals receiving basic immunosuppression, only mild (A_{0-1} or A_1) or moderate (A_2) grades of rejection were observed (Tables 3, 15). Severe rejection in the initial biopsy was not seen in these patients nor in these experimental animals. This was certainly not the case in those animals not receiving basic immunosuppression (Table 1 and Fig. 6).

In assessing the relevance of histological findings, we must consider if the material obtained from a single biopsy is representative of the changes in the whole liver. In general, a core biopsy is performed from the right lateral liver lobe of the patients. In the animals relatively less material from the right liver area was available. When the liver was prepared and assessed in layers in the postmortem histology a surprising heterogeneity of the findings was noted (Fig. 5a). This heterogeneity was more extensive the more rapidly developing and more severe the rejection. In two animals not receiving basic immunosuppression and after particularly severe rejection and death at the end of the first week, there was a wide range of histologic findings: areas of both severe and mild rejection (Fig. 5a and 5b) representing a heterogeneity over more than two grades. However, this was exceptional. At the end of long courses of acute rejection, no heterogeneity was detectable. In animals who died within the first three postoperative weeks, grade A_3 predominated but there were several areas of grade A_2 rejection.

For practical purposes it can be assumed that under basic immunosuppression and after longer courses of acute rejection, histologic changes within the liver will be uniform throughout. Only with very early or very severe rejection or under conditions in which the basic immunosuppression is stopped altogether or reduced for clinical reasons, will the histologic findings be heterogeneous.

Pathophysiologically, however, it is especially important and interesting that the liver does not react homogeneously to all disorders. Some areas seem to be severely damaged, other areas only slightly. The reasons are unknown. Perhaps one explanation is the variety of presentations of offending substances, elements etc. Another explanation may be that defense mechanisms are variously available or effective in the regions of the liver. Several factors may play a role, e.g., the experimentally (Groth 1968) as well as the clinically well-known decrease in liver blood flow with rejection (Pichlmayr 1983, Merion 1988), regional disorders of liver blood flow in conjunction with tissue edema or regional pressure conditions similar to the situation in the Budd-Chiari syndrome in which an especially marked increase of the size of the caudate lobe is known, or the compensatory effect of the dual blood supply of the liver. The assessment of such pathogenic mechanisms, however, was not the aim of this study. Nevertheless the existence of heterogeneity in the liver is relevant for clinical decision-making regarding rejection. This corresponds to the heterogeneity of rejection findings in heart transplantation. In heart transplantation several biopsies are *always* necessary for the determination of acute rejection, and, these biopsies have to be taken from various regions of the heart (Haverich 1984, Westra 1987, Kemnitz 1992). In liver transplantation this heterogeneity requires, additionally, that decisions regarding treatment of rejection only be made in the context of the clinical picture. Nevertheless, the question remains: Why with homogeneous blood flow through the whole liver and with homogeneously distributed immunosuppressive agents, slight homogeneous changes of the whole organ are not reversible without additional rejection treatment. Obviously there *are* differences between the clinically symptomatic and the asymptomatic findings of A_{0-1} or A_1. Perhaps they cannot be detected by histology. Perhaps these differences have an immunologic etiology.

In this context it is especially interesting that in a study on spontaneous tolerance after liver transplantation done by Engemann in rats (Engemann 1985) tolerant donor-recipient combinations with long-term survival without basic immunosuppression revealed extensive histological signs consistent with acute rejection. Engemann confirmed in this very detailed and exact immunological study what had been described by other groups. Starzl found in 1965 infiltrates of the liver graft with mononuclear cells independent of rejection in dogs. Similar findings were obtained later by others in rats (Zimmermann 1982, Kamada 1983). In the present study these findings can be confirmed for the human as well.

The pathophysiological interpretation of these early postoperative histological "patterns of rejection" have not become easier by these experimental and clinical findings. Besides the pure processes of rejection obviously other pathogeneic mechanisms must be considered as well. Independent from the various theories and interpretations about the development of the histological findings, three different constellations with different prognoses can be discerned concerning the clinical relevance of the histological findings:

1. In the postoperative period histological findings consistent with mild acute rejection without a clinical picture of rejection must be considered standard. It does not require specific treatment as long as basic immunosuppression is instituted.

2. Histological grades A_{0-1} or A_1 in conjunction with a clinical picture of rejection requires immediate treatment for rejection in order to avert progression of graft dysfunction.

3. Histological evidence of moderate acute rejection in conjunction with a corresponding clinical picture of rejection requires immediate and especially highly potent treatment at the outset. This should include mono- or polyclonal antibodies. One must recognize that the process may already be irreversible and that retransplantation, in spite of the highly potent therapy, may be required.

FREQUENCY OF ACUTE REJECTION

Sixty-one percent of all patients observed over six months suffered acute rejection within the first three postoperative weeks after liver transplantation. A larger group of patients observed for three postoperative weeks had a frequency of acute rejection of 65%. For the purposes of this discussion, the larger group of patients will be used. The frequency of about 60% corresponds to the findings of other groups (Kirby 1987, Pichlmayr—overview 1987b, Ascher 1988, Porter 1988, Munn 1988, Klintmalm 1989 and 1991) and it corresponds to our own experimental findings in the small group of animals under basic immunosuppression (62.5%/27.8-86.3).[B] These animals developed clinical and histological evidence of acute rejection (Fig. 9).

This high frequency of acute rejection contradicts the privileged immunological status of the liver. This brings up two questions regarding acute rejection:

1. What are the potential risk factors for early postoperative rejection?

2. What are the features of acute rejection?

POTENTIAL RISK FACTORS FOR THE DEVELOPMENT OF ACUTE REJECTION

Risk factors can be of very different origin. Three factors must be considered:

1. The condition of the recipient just prior to transplantation.

2. The quality of the donor organ.

3. The whole clinical picture in the early postoperative period and its effects on the graft and the recipient.

Concerning 1: *Patients with liver cirrhosis suffered acute rejections more frequently after liver transplantation than other patients.* In contrast to this, the kind of basic disease—whether it is benign or malignant—plays no role.

The statistical significance between the cirrhotic and the noncirrhotic condition is especially revealing in the patients with malignant tumors (Table 10d). Even after applying Yates' correction (Yates 1980) for small or imbalanced samples, the comparison reveals a highly significant value of $chi^2_y = 7.02$ and a likelihood of error $\alpha < 1\%$. In this group of patients the cirrhosis seems to predominate. This group of patients is composed only of patients in very poor general conditions. The question, however, is why the general condition of the recipient *prior to* transplantation should have any influence on the immunological process *after* transplantation. This most likely has to do with a general—as opposed to a specific— effect, when a complicated or critical condition causes or favors further complications. This corresponds to conventional wisdom and to statistical results after liver transplantation indicating that the chance for survival depends on the preoperative status of the recipient. Especially with regard to cirrhotic diseases, Lauchart demonstrated that the status of the recipient is directly related to early postoperative mortality (Lauchart 1986). Since acute rejection plays such a large role in the early postoperative period, it is easily conceivable that there is a nonspecific relationship between the cirrhotic condition and the frequency of rejection.

Concerning 2: *Acute rejection is more likely to occur in severely damaged grafts than in undamaged grafts.* "Graft damage" is a general term for which there is no objective criteria. Yet it is useful. An increase in transaminases of more than twice the median peak level of all patients just after the transplantation has proven to be valuable in assessing graft damage. It was used in other studies on the early graft function (Gubernatis 1988b, Gubernatis 1989a) and will serve as the limiting value for the purposes of this discussion.

The influence of severe graft damage on the frequency of rejection is statistically significant ($\alpha = 4\%$). The likelihood of error corrected according to Yates is $\alpha_y = 7.8\%$ and is therefore slightly above the generally accepted level of significance. However, the Yates-correction was only applied because the distribution is unbalanced and not because of the small sample size.

In this context it should be mentioned that the more frequent occurrence of acute rejection after severe graft damage is not an artifact caused by the changes of the morphology, such as a so-called harvesting lesion. The diagnosis of acute rejection is not only based on morphological but also on clinical considerations in conjunction with the histology, and the histological signs of rejection are different from those of graft damage. However, it is possible that large areas of necrosis secondary to severe graft damage could be misinterpreted histologically as rejection. The question is whether or not a histologic grade of A_2 in a damaged graft is due predominantly to that preexisting damage or to acute rejection.

In conjunction with the significantly more frequent occurrence of rejection after severe graft damage the nonsignificantly more frequent finding of A_1 has to be considered exclusively due to rejection which must be treated promptly and aggressively.

Concerning 3: *The whole clinical situation in the immediate postoperative period has no influence on the frequency of acute rejection which could be assessed by the parameter "basic immunosuppression".*

If the graft functions well and the recipient is in good condition, standard immunosuppression consisting of cyclosporin A and prednisone can be administered. If graft function is decreased and is insufficient to metabolize cyclosporin or if the recipient is in a critical situation, an individualized immunosuppressive regimen will be initiated independent of the cause for the dysfunction. In this case triple or quadruple drug combinations are used with low dosages of each drug and cyclosporin is sometimes withdrawn (Pichlmayr 1987a). As seen in Table 12 there is no difference in the frequency of acute rejections between the patients with standard and the patients with individualized immunosuppression.

Of course the patient's early postoperative condition is a result of graft quality as well as his condition prior to the operation. However, these are not the only important considerations in the early postoperative period. Yet whatever the considerations, acute rejection often can be averted by basic immunosuppression and when it occurs treatment can be individualized.

FEATURES OF ACUTE REJECTION

The time of onset of acute rejection is generally consistent: *Most acute rejections occurs between postoperative day 5 and 8, mostly on day 5 or 6.*

Although the early onset is surprising, it is confirmed by the animal studies. Animals receiving basic immunosuppression manifested signs of rejection on day 7. Animals without basic immunosuppression suffered lethal acute rejections and died on postoperative days 6 or 7 (median day 6). This means, that the rejection process in these animals had already begun. Basic immunosuppression may therefore not only lead to less frequent and less severe acute rejection but also to a delay in onset. The findings in animals not receiving basic immunosuppression corresponds to the clinical situation in which potent immunosuppression cannot be instituted because of special clinical considerations (Pichlmayr 1987a) or in situations in which the immunological risk is high, e.g., in strongly reacting donor-recipient combinations.

The experimental and clinical data reveal that as early as postoperative days 4-5 one must be alert for the manifestations of acute rejection.

There is no aspect of the presentation that is pathognomonic. On the contrary there is a high degree of variability. Early in the course not all classic symptoms are yet present. The experimental and clinical data are consistent in this regard. The diversity of presentation is not new. It is noted in various publications investigating other phenomena in conjunction with rejection. The first publication concerning the clinical aspects of rejection (Pichlmayr 1983) describes a variety of presentations. It indicated there was no single classical sign of rejection. Therefore one must not wait for the full-blown picture of rejection before making the diagnosis. For example, an increase in bilirubin can be an expression of cyclosporin A toxicity, but waiting for a cyclosporin blood level unnecessarily delays the prompt diagnosis and treatment of rejection. In this regard the treatment in the patient illustrated in Figure 25 could have been treated one day earlier if the increase in bilirubin would have been considered a sign of rejection. Such considerations are also relevant to the early recognition of repeated rejection episodes.

The histological features of acute rejection have been described in detail in accord with the so-called Hannover Classification (Kemnitz

1986, 1989a, b, 1991). It is remarkable that the combination of acute rejection and concomitant cholangitis was only seen in conjunction with type II.

Two clinical-histological patterns of acute rejection can be distinguished: type I includes an increase in transaminases sometimes combined with cholestasis and type II includes an increase in bilirubin and fever frequently combined with cholestasis and cholangitis. In addition, combinations of types I and II exist. Only when this occurs, can virtually the entire "classic" picture of acute rejection be seen.

Interestingly, cholestasis is present in both types I and II—even in animals with basic immunosuppression, but it is absent in animals without immunosuppression. It is tempting to consider that perhaps cholestasis is somehow related to immunosuppression. However, cholestasis is absent in most patients without rejection *who are receiving basic immunosuppression.* Perhaps the phenomenon of cholestasis is due to the hepatotoxicity of immunosuppression complicated by acute rejection, a condition characterized by decreased hepatocellular function and increased sensitivity to toxic substances. In any case, cholestasis as such is therefore not pathonogmonic of rejection.

The same is true of the noninfectious cholangitis. When it is associated with rejection, it may be due to the de novo expression of donor MHC antigens on the bile ducts which is especially strong in early after transplantation (Steiniger 1984, Steinhoff 1988a,b, Steinhoff 1990c) and which causes a corresponding recipient reaction. There are various observationss in the literature concerning changes in the bile duct epithelium with rejection alone and in conjunction with cholestasis and cholangitis (Hunt 1967, Öhler 1972, Kamada 1983, Engemann 1985). However, these findings derive partly from nonphysiological models of liver transplantation without reconstruction of arterial blood supply. In such models, even in syngeneic combinations, pathological changes in the bile ducts were observed (Kamada 1983). In this regard our experimental findings concerning the considerable vascular changes early after liver transplantation as a sign of early rejection may be relevant. These changes were seen especially in animals not receiving immunosuppression, whereas in animals receiving basic immunosuppression such changes were seen later and were less pronounced. In humans these changes are seen in conjunction with chronic processes (Vierling 1985, Gront 1986, Kemnitz 1989a and b). Animals not receiving immunosuppression demonstrate clearly that such vascular changes are also possible in conjunction with acute rejection in the early postoperative phase. In these animals there was neither cholestasis nor cholangitis, in contrast to the immunosuppressed animal group. This means that vascular changes might contribute to deterioration of the bile ducts, however, they play neither the only nor the decisive role in this process. Other, more decisive mechanisms must be present such as the special location of dendritic cells around the bile ducts (Steiniger 1984) or the strong de novo expression of MHC antigens on bile duct membranes. An additive effect of various mechanisms could explain why cholestasis occurs in both rejection patterns type I and II with a stronger expression in type II, whereas cholangitis is seen only in conjunction with type II. In this regard immunological factors and therefore HLA-compatibility are especially relevant.

INFLUENCE OF HLA-COMPATIBILITY ON ACUTE REJECTION

HLA-compatibility has a considerable influence on acute rejection. Patients with one compatibility on the HLA-DR locus most frequently express type I rejection with an increase in transaminases and sometimes cholestasis. Patients with no compatibility on the HLA-DR locus express type II rejection with an increase in bilirubin and fever frequently in combination with severe cholestasis and noninfectious cholangitis or the mixed type I and II with features of type II predominating.

These observations are important for early diagnosis and for understanding pathogenesis. However, the investigation could only be performed in patients with no and one DR compatibility, because no patients with other compatibilities were available.

Knowledge of HLA-compatibility is especially important for early recognition of an ongoing rejection. Incompatibility should create a high level of suspicion for rejection. A certain characteristic pattern of rejection can be expected not only with recurrent rejection but also for the first rejection if the individual HLA-compatibility is known (Gubernatis 1988d, e, 1989).

In the experimental part of this study, the influence of DR-compatibility on rejection was noted. However, the less frequent observations and blood samplings etc. limited systematic investigations. Furthermore the investigations were limited as follows: two animal donors were DR homozygous and in four animals only one DR locus could be determined.

In contrast to HLA-DR-compatibility no influence on rejection could be detected for the HLA-A and -B loci. This is especially interesting with regard to pathogenesis. It can be guessed that the causes already mentioned, especially the de novo expression of class II antigens after liver transplantation (Steinhoff 1988a and 1991) may play the decisive role in rejection. The development of cholestasis expressed in both types I and II— but especially strongly only in type II—could be caused by completely different immunological mechanisms such as vascular problems in conjunction with antibody-mediated reactivity and cellular aggression against bile duct epithelia. In particular, the antibody-mediated assault against the vessel wall in acute rejection after liver transplantation is derived from experience with chronic rejection, with kidney transplantation and new clinical knowledge regarding hyperacute rejection.

Cholangitis is associated with an especially strong expression of DR antigens on bile duct epithelia (Steinhoff 1988a). On the other hand, cholangitis was limited in situations with complete DR mismatches, and it would therefore be observed only in type II. Other bile duct-specific antigens could play a similar role in primary biliary cirrhosis (Neuberger 1982). This, however, is a hypothesis derived by comparison to changes in chronic rejection in conjunction with chronic destructive cholangitis (Öhlert 1972), i.e., by comparison with the vanishing bile duct syndrome. With regard to the vanishing bile duct syndrome and HLA-DR-compatibility, a controversial association was observed (Donaldson 1987, Markus 1987) in long-term liver transplant survivors in Pittsburgh: the better the HLA-DR-compatibility the worse the survival rate. This surprising result has just been confirmed in principle by White who performed a similar study on Pittsburgh's patients during a later time period (White in press). The studies were performed independently from each other, and the situation became confused and controversial the last few years. In further analyses and studies all other potential factors and causes of graft loss have to be considered. Initial nonfunction, technical and vascular problems, exacerbation of preexisting infections, complications associated with blood loss and many other factors may overwhelm the influence of immunological factors on the survival. The relationship between long-term survival and HLA-compatibility can only be assessed with regard to the whole postoperative course in a very large number of patients.

For this reason such an analysis was not performed in this study:

Our findings do not reveal any relationship between HLA-compatibility and the frequency of acute rejection.

For this reason the liver transplantation centers of Cambridge (Sir R. Calne), London (R. Williams), Paris (H. Bismuth) and Hannover (R. Pichlmayr) in conjunction with Eurotransplant in Leiden (G. Persijn) established a combined study named L'ESPRIT (Liver: European Study Protocol for the Relevance of Immunology in Transplantation) in order to investigate the influence of HLA-compatibility on patient survival with regard to all potentially significant factors as mentioned above. We are just in the process of analyzing our data obtained from 549 patients receiving first grafts with an overall one-year graft survival of 70.4%. A beneficial effect of HLA-B-compatibility on one-year graft survival can be detected in contrast to the HLA-A mismatch groups in which no effect can be observed. Surprisingly HLA-DR compatibility seems to be detrimental to graft survival. As yet, this result is not completely

significant; however, it is quite consistent with the findings of the other authors mentioned above. The first few results are in press (Thorogood in press).

Concerning donor-recipient-allocation, the HLA-compatibility has no influence on the decision-making as yet.

TREATMENT AND PROGNOSIS OF ACUTE REJECTION

Most acute rejections can be treated successfully by bolus injections of steroids. Three bolus injections daily are adequate in general. In some patients up to five bolus injections were necessary, yet sometimes only 1-2 boluses were sufficient. Some question whether rejection reversed by a single steroid bolus should, in fact, have been treated at all. We believe that treatment in this circumstance is justified since even mild histological and clinical findings of acute rejection can be the harbinger of the full-blown picture. On the other hand, single or double bolus injections are rare.

All rejection episodes that do not progress after treatment and therefore do not require retransplantation or result in death were considered reversible. The clinical and histological signs became normal promptly with the exception of the findings of cholangitis and cholestasis which persist for a considerable time after other parameters have corrected. This also stresses the theory of the additional and different pathomechanisms of its development. There is a group of indirect treatment failures, i.e., those patients initially treated successfully for rejection but who die from a nontreatable infection which arose as a direct result of the rejection treatment. Such infections have occurred after only steroid therapy was prescribed without any other special drugs. Steroid-treated rejections fail in only 14% of cases. This good result not only holds for patients receiving the general regimen of basic immunosuppression; it is true as well in patients receiving individualized basic immunosuppression. In these cases immunosuppression was modified for various reasons. Dosages were low in order to avoid toxicity; an increased risk of rejection was therefore accepted. Statistically no increase in the frequency of rejection could be detected in this group as already mentioned above (Table 12). Concerning the severity of rejections (Table 13), these are more severe. However, the difference is not significant. This indicates that rejections that occur in patients receiving individualized basic immunosuppression are comparable to rejections occurring in standard situations.

Severe clinical rejection was treated with poly- or monoclonal antibodies in addition to steroids and had a poor prognosis with regard to both rejection and lethal infection. In this study irreversibe rejection had to be expected in 50% of the cases, and lethal infectious complications comprised 64% of these treatment failures. Comparison with the group of steroid-only treated patients is highly significant (α <1%). However, this is certainly not surprising as it concerns two different risk groups.

Of course, this does not demonstrate that antibodies are less effective than steroid-only treatment. It indicates that in spite of potent antibody treatment a considerable number of irreversible rejections nevertheless have to be expected. A further increase in dosage or duration of antibody treatment is not reasonable due to the risk of lethal infections. Perhaps this would decrease irreversible rejections, but the price would be high since lethal infections would increase. Our poor results in treatment of severe rejection corresponds to results in the literature if patients are assessed by risk groups. For example, Wood distinguishes four risk groups (Wood 1988). When monoclonal antibodies are employed as rescue therapy, rejection is irreversible in 50% of cases which corresponds exactly to our results. Wood also described fulminant fatal infections, in part after retransplantation performed after unsuccessful antirejection treatment. Other authors have obtained much better results. Colonna achieved complete remission in 14 out of 25 patients (Colonna 1987), and only some patients had to be retransplanted. Delmonico had a treatment failure rate of 30%, and he retransplanted only 4% of patients (Delmonico 1988). Klintmalm had a good primary success rate, but saw a considerably increasing number of infections, lymphomas and deaths (Klintmalm

1991). This brings up the questions: When is rejection considered steroid-resistant and when should antibody therapy be instituted? This is a question whether or not the risk groups are comparable. Our results in treating steroid-resistant patients are with polyclonal antibodies in contrast to the patients in the literature who were mostly treated with the monoclonal antibody OKT3. Monoclonal antibody success rates seem to be better, even if there is as yet "not enough convincing evidence that they are superior to polyclonals" (Land 1991). In the future it can be expected that with the development of new monoclonal antibodies (Land 1991) the success rate in every respect will increase (direct effect on rejection signs, indirect effect on later lethal infections). Nevertheless, the clinical decision regarding the use of mono- or polyclonal antibodies must take into account the considerable failure rate and factors regarding retransplantation. The failure rate of retransplantation, depending on the indication, is high in the case of irreversible acute rejection with one-year survival rates of about 35% (Starzl 1985, Shaw 1985a, Shaw 1985b) up to 55% (Morel 1991). However, if retransplantation is performed electively results are comparable to those obtained with first grafts. Mora and Klintmalm (Mora 1990) therefore decided to treat severe rejection early on by retransplantation instead of by repeated attempts with medical therapies (Klintmalm 1991).

In all cases of rejection therapy when poly- or monoclonal antibodies are necessary one has to expect high failure rates and the indications for retransplantation should be established from the outset.

Can patients at high risk for irreversible rejection be identified clinically? Histological findings can be helpful The severity detected in the initial biopsy has proven to be of predictive value. As shown in Table 23 most rejection grades A_{0-1} or A_1 can be treated by steroids only in contrast to grade A_2 which frequently requires antibodies. Of course, this is only a relative statement, but histology can be important in prompt diagnosis and treatment. For example, in two patients grade A_1 was seen in the first biopsy. The patients were not treated, and according to the definition, this was not considered rejection. Later, in both patients grade A_2 was observed and they were successfully treated only with steroids alone. This means that the rejection was less severe than in patients with grade A_2 histology on initial biopsy! This example supports the above mentioned considerations on the predictive value of the initial biopsy. This result is supported by recent findings of McDonald (McDonald 1989) in a smaller number of patients revealing a high percentage of steroid-resistant rejections in patients with manifestations of moderate rejection on initial biopsy whereas those with only mild rejection could generally be treated successfully with steroids only.

The following conclusions can be drawn: The initial biopsy provides a good prediction of eventual outcome. This means that in patients with only mild symptoms and signs of rejection histological findings of severe rejection represents a poor prognostic. If potent treatment fails retransplantation should be considered early.

The clinical patterns were also assessed regarding their predictive value. Type I seems to be more easily treatable. However, it was followed by more recurrent rejections. The reason cannot be inadequate rejection therapy because complete remission of rejection occurred in all patients. The findings are therefore moot. An influence of the clinical pattern on the response to therapy cannot be determined, at least not for the patients in this study. Also, HLA-compatibility did not have any influence on the effectiveness of rejection treatment in this study.

In conclusion, aside from the histological grade of severity in the initial biopsy there was no parameter of predictive value. Which patient will suffer rejection, in whom this will be irreversible, in whom therapy will be effective and who will remain free from recurrent rejection cannot be predicted. In the future immunological parameters for predicting rejection, response to treatment, and spontaneous or induced tolerance will probably be available (Calne 1991).

In this study, of all patients in whom acute rejection in the early postoperative period was suc- *cessfully treated no further rejection occurred in 56%. The remainder, 44%, underwent recurrent acute or chronic rejection. Patients without any signs of rejection in the early postoperative period remained free from acute rejection in the long-term.*

COURSE WITHOUT AND AFTER CESSATION OF BASIC IMMUNO-SUPPRESSION AND TOLERANCE

The animals without basic immunosuppression can be divided into two gropus. In one group animals died early postoperatively (median day 6) from severe rejection. In the other group animals survived this phase and died later (median day 40, longest survival 116 days) from rejection. No animal survived without basic immunosuppression. Consequently neither the results of Myburgh (Myburgh 1975, Myburgh 1980) nor the findings of Engemann (Engemann 1985) can be confirmed. In Myburgh's experience all animals of the same species as used in this study (monkeys) died early postoperatively from irreversible rejection (survival 13 ± 3 days, no longer survival). Engemann achieved long-term survival without basic immunosuppression in rats but only in special genetically defined donor-recipient combinations. But even in these so-called "tolerant" stem combinations, Engemann described histopathological findings consistent with rejection. This is consistent with early findings of Starzl in dogs(Kukral 1966). He observed in all animals, independently from the clinical occurrence of rejection, histological signs of rejection. Also in this study several animals survived for a long-term. Starzl explained such findings later by better compatibility in these surviving donor-recipient combinations (Starzl 1969). In pigs longer survival without immunosuppression could be achieved (Calne 1969b); in some animals survival times of more than 100 days were observed and Bockhorn demonstrated a clear relationship between survival time and compatibility in the SLA system and the MHC system of the pig (Bockhorn 1975). Our findings concerning histocompatibility, including DR-typing, neither confirmed nor refuted these results due to the unbalanced sample survey. Engemann explained the longer survival by invoking the development of tolerance, and he considered the morphological signs consistent with rejection an expression of the recipient's reaction with the donor antigens. Moreover, he stated that this is immunologically necessary for the development of tolerance and only a situation without any immunosuppression can lead to tolerance.

The same mechanism of the development of tolerance should be responsible for the longer survival after cessation of immunosuppression, and Engemann and other researchers detected the same morphological signs as in acute rejection. In these cases the type of tolerance is not the classical neonatal type that occurs by deletion. It is a functional reactive type based on partial suppression. This can only partly be supported by our experimental and clinical findings. The experimental data revealed a longer survival even after the onset of rejection; however, this never led to complete remission. The whole picture is therefore consistent with more or less strongly expressed rejection. In 20% of patients, there were histological signs of mild rejection without clinical symptoms. According to the theories mentioned above this could be the mechanism of development of tolerance. However, the question remains why the other 20% of patients did not suffer rejection nor develop tolerance. For the development of tolerance a phase without any immunosuppression is thought to be required although cyclosporin A is considered to act as an inducer (Engemann 1985). Our experimental results cannot confirm this.

All animals in which immunosuppression was stopped developed rejection. However, the time varied and most of the animals survived longer than 100 days after cessation of cyclosporin A—up to 481 days. Animals receiving monoclonal antibodies (Steinhoff 1990a) and animals in which basic immunosuppression was stopped only in the later postoperative course (day 191 and 192) survived especially long. As all of these animals eventually developed rejection, it seems to be more a question of terminology whether longer survival is described as delayed recognition of alloantigens and delayed onset of rejection or as development of functional tolerance with partial suppression. A specific inductive effect seems not to be present because the delayed onset of rejection is not only seen after cyclosporin A or monoclonal antibodies but was also described by Starzl in dogs after cessation of azathioprine (Starzl 1965). The findings of the experimental results of the spontaneous course and the course after cessation of basic immunosuppression are as follows:

Adequate basic immunosuppression is especially important in the early phase after liver transplantation. Otherwise severe rejection will invariably develop rapidly and be irreversible. In the longer term, basic immunosuppression is generally necessary or rejection will ensue. Short-term cessation of basic immunosuppression later in the course, however, is possible, and the risk of the rapid development of rejection is low. Cessation of basic immunosuppression to enable the recipient to react with the donor antigens to induce partial tolerance is not indicated—at least for the time being—as such "tolerance" cannot be achieved reliably and is always, as demonstrated above, followed by rejection in the longer term.

HYPERACUTE REJECTION

In both the experimental and the clinical studies it could be demonstrated that hyperacute rejection after liver transplantation exists.

This was surprising because it was long believed from both experimental data (Starzl 1969, Calne 1969a,b, Kamada 1981, Houssin 1985) and clinical observations (Starzl 1974, Calne 1979) that the liver is resistant to antibody-mediated rejection.

Animals sensitized by donor blood and skin had remarkably shorter survival in most cases; most died immediately after the operation. The operation itself was performed in all cases without any problems, reperfusion was immediate and homogeneous and thorough perioperative monitoring did not reveal any indication of a nonimmunological cause of early graft failure. The influence and the relevance of immunological causes for the early graft failure were obtained from histological findings. Animals that died immediately postoperatively had hemorrhagic necrosis on the postmortem examination (Fig. 11a) and massive deposits of fibrinogen and immunoglobulins (Fig. 11b). In one of these animals the surface of the liver suddenly became marbled after initial homogeneous reperfusion (Fig. 10). In this case the histological findings could already be detected in the intraoperative biopsy. The clinical and histological picture in these animals is consistent with hyperacute rejection. Our experimental results (Gubernatis 1987) correspond to the findings of Knechtle (Knechtle 1987a and b) who demonstrated the existence of hyperacute rejection after liver transplantation in an experimental model as well. He performed the classical "antibody transfer" experiment in rats, and in this immunologically defined model he demonstrated hyperacute rejection definitely. However, this antibody transfer experiment is not feasible in primates: on the one hand no in-bred stems are available and on the other hand the number of animals required to obtain an adequate sample of antibodies—which means the number of animals that had to be specifically sensitized and sacrificed afterwards—would be too high. Furthermore the reaction of the recipients varied widely, as with humans. One animal died on postoperative day 7 with histological evidence of hemorrhage and very severe cellular rejection. A second animal survived until postoperative day 22 and died from severe acute rejection grade A_3, quite similar to other animals without basic immunosuppression but without specific presensitization.

The resulting question from these data that cannot be answered at thismoment is not why hyperacute rejection occurs in the liver, but why hyperacute rejection does not occur in all cases of existing donor-specific presensitization. The same mechanisms could be responsible that have been discussed as possible causes for the immunologically privileged status of the liver. The vessel structures of the liver display HLA class I antigens (Daar 1984) and are therefore a major target in antibody-mediated rejection. Because of the dual blood supply, occlusion in one system is compensated by the other system. Ischemic necrosis is prevented in this way. In the sinusoids the endothelial windows are widely spaced and basal membranes are absent which may play a role in the aggregation of platelets. The liver releases soluble class I antigens

which may lead to the neutralization of specific antibodies (Kamada 1985). The presence of Kupffer's cells as part of the RES and the fact that circulating immune complexes can be cleared may play a role. Finally the absolute size of the liver and the ratio of antigens to antibodies could have an influence.

These mechanisms may be the reason for the great variability of clinical appearance and may be responsible for the fact that in the human no hyperacute rejection was observed for a long time. Even recentlys only isolated cases have been observed. Two features play a special role.

One main problem is the distinction between immunological and nonimmunological causes of early graft failure. Of course, a rapid and severe immunological reaction can cause graft failure at the outset of reperfusion, and Starzl explains at least a part of the nonfunctioning organs on the basis of immunological considerations. Nevertheless it is helpful and in this study a prerequisite for establishing the diagnosis of hyperacute rejection if at least a very short period of initial graft function occurs. General parameters such as the onset of bile production, production of clotting factors, decrease in lactate and similar criteria that distinguish reversible and irreversible graft damage (Gubernatis 1988a and b, Gubernatis 1989a) are inadequate indicators of the classical appearance of hyperacute rejection. As yet only the measurement of total oxygen consumption can reliably detect even a short period of initial function after reperfusion (Bornscheuer 1988, Gubernatis 1989b), as it is demonstrated in the first patient. In this patient signs of an immunological reaction could already be seen in the histological specimen taken at the end of operation, and the biopsy taken 24 hours after reperfusion revealed massive deposits of immunoglobulins and fibrinogen. Clinically this course would have shown the typical signs of an initial nonfunction if the measurements mentioned had not been performed.

The second problem is the variable appearance of antibody-mediated rejection (Gubernatis 1989d). In addition to the classical "immediate type", there seems to be a "delayed type" that occurs after a few days.

This delayed type was observed by the transplant groups of McMaster and Calne (personal communications, and Huebscher 1989, Bird 1989). The patients had a well functioning graft and had no postoperative problems until days 2 or 3 when suddenly a severe graft deterioration occurred and no other reasons than an immunological one could be detected. The patients were retransplanted and the first grafts showed a dark discolored surface. Intrahepatically disseminated intravascular thrombosis was present whereas the extrahepatic vessels were patent. In our experience the second patient is an example of a course that is consistent with so-called accelerated rejection. However, due to the histological findings including massive immunoglobulin deposits it has to be considered hyperacute antibody-mediated rejection. In all patients with the so-called delayed type rejection initial graft function could clearly be demonstrated by classical parameters although the onset of graft deterioration was delayed. This may be the reason why in most the clinical cases this type has not been observed.

ADDENDUM

Developments to improve the operative technique in the animal model

Besides the standardization of the technique as one of the presuppositions for a rapid and simultaneously thorough and safe operative procedure some special details of the operative technique were changed. Some especially relevant developments are described here.

1. Anastomosis of the bile ducts

Anastomosis of the bile ducts was done in a long (circa 1 cm) side-to-side manner. This technique was developed by Neuhaus in pigs, and he introduced this technique for Rhesus monkeys as well (Neuhaus 1982). By means of a careful no-touch technique preserving all the tissue between the hepatic artery and the common bile duct in the donor as well as in the recipient, problems caused by inadequate blood flow to the distal bile ducts were not observed. Due to the size of the anastomosis, stenoses—even a functional,

temporary one causing postoperative swelling or edema, are very unlikely and were not seen in this study. Anastomoses were sutured using PDS 6/0 BV 1. No leakage was observed. Thus the good results obtained by Neuhaus when he introduced this technique can be confirmed for all the transplantations performed during this study.

2. Anastomosis of the hepatic artery

For reconstruction of the artery either the celiac trunk including an aortic patch is anastomosed onto the recipient aorta in a subdiaphragmatic position or the celiac trunk is anastomosed onto the aorta below the branching of the renal vessels using a long aortic conduit. The second technique has become the preferred one. In order to facilitate blood flow and to avoid disturbances where the celiac trunk branches from the donor aorta in a nearly right angle the aorta distal to the take-off is sutured with "6.0-prolene" to form a conical vessel. The thoracic segment of the aorta (which is the conduit) is turned about a sagittal axis from the thoracic to the abdominal position, but exactly at the level of the recipient thus carefully avoiding twisting of the vessel in its own axis. The right colonic flexure must be dissected a little. The artery should finally be situated dorsal to the portal vein, i.e., to the new hepatoduodenal ligament. At the end of the procedure the hepatic artery must have enough space to lay without tension in spite of the relatively strong and rigid aortic conduit. For the same reason all tissue has to be removed from the small hepatic artery during the donor organ preparation and longer ligatures have to be avoided because both could turn and twist the vessel and prevent the artery from finding its own optimal position which would inevitably lead to thrombosis. A major advantage of the conduit anastomosed on the infrarenal abdominal aorta is that this anastomosis can be performed after reperfusion without interfering, i.e., reducing the flow of the portal vein, as the supramesenteric. The proximal aorta is open during throughout the procedure. Thrombosis of the aortic conduit did not occur. In all postmortem examinations the hepatic artery was patent.

3. Relevance of the surgical management of the retroperitoneum

The retroperitoneum was never unnecessarily opened. However, in the area of the suprarenal gland an incision of the retroperitoneum is unavoidable. This area was oversewn during the anhepatic phase using very fine prolene sutures. It is important that the edges of the retroperitoneal incision are not widely or roughly sutured. Large sutures through the muscles or the suprarenal gland would cause new hemorrhage. Compression cannot be achieved by such sutures, and bleeding would continue beneath the sutures without being visible or controllable. Evaluation of the integrity of the retroperitoneal surface during the hepatectomy and the exact surgical treatment during the anhepatic phase are two of the most important considerations for the prevention of bleeding after reperfusion.

EARLY POSTOPERATIVE REJECTION AFTER LIVER TRANSPLANTATION

This is a combined experimental and clinical study on the early postoperative rejection in liver grafts, the relevance, the possibility of diagnosis-making, the requirements for therapy, the prognosis, the efficiency of various treatments and the influence of the different grades of immunological compatibility.

In the experimental part 47 orthotopic liver transplantations were performed in Rhesus monkeys and findings concerning the spontaneous course, the course under basic immunosuppression and after cessation of immunosuppression were analyzed. Furthermore one group of animals was donor-specifically presensitized.

In the clinical part 81 consecutively liver grafted patients were observed prior to, during and continuously over six months after transplantation of until death and all findings were assessed concerning the diagnosis and therapy of rejection and the differentiation from other causes of graft deterioration.

IN THE EXPERIMENTAL PART THE FOLLOWING MAIN RESULTS CAN BE OBTAINED:

• All animals without immunosuppression experience a rejection independent from whether they never receive immunosuppression or their initially applied basic immunosuppression is cessated later. The development of rejection is more rapid early postoperatively compared with the situation after cessation of immunosuppression in a later postoperative phase. Rejection is not inevitably leading to death in all cases just after the onset. Animals surviving the initial phase of rejection show permanent signs of rejection in a changing intensity but they never show complete remission. Finally all animals die by rejection (longest survival 116 days), no animal develops a permanent tolerance.

• Under the experimental condition without applying immunosuppression the clinical and histological signs of rejection consistent with the signs in the human situation could be observed and investigated in a much more distinctive expression.

• The especially predominant histological findings under the situation without immunosuppression represent a valuable material for the consideration of histological findings in humans. By such a comparison the especially strong appearance of vascular changes already in the early phase after transplantation and the absence of severe cholestasis in the experimental model is especially remarkable.

• By a donor-specific presensitization the existence of hyperacute rejection after liver transplantation could be demonstrated for the first time in the closely human-related Rhesus monkey model.

IN THE CLINICAL PART THE FOLLOWING MAIN RESULTS CAN BE OBTAINED:

• There is no single finding of parameter that is pathognomonic for a treatment-requiring rejection alone.

• 80% of the patients reveal histological signs of rejection in the early postoperative phase. Without simultaneous clinical signs these findings are spontaneously reversible under basic immunosuppression (without special rejection treatment).

• 60% of the patients experience a treatment-requiring rejection in the early postoperative phase. The onset of the first treatment-requiring day is the fifth to the eighth postoperative day in most cases.

• Rejections occur more likely in patients with a preoperatively severe cirrhotic condition and in patients receiving a damaged, badly functioning graft.

• Two features of acute rejection with different clinical appearance can be differentiated. The patterns individually remain the same ones in case of recurrent rejections.

• Most of the rejections could be successfully treated by three bolus applications of 500 mg methylprednisolone each. In case of more severe rejections requiring additional application of poly- or monoclonal antibodies a high failure rate (circa 50-60% in this study) should be expected and the indication for retransplantation should be considered in time.

• After successfully treated first rejection most of the patients remain free from rejection in the further course.

• In case no rejection occurs in the early postoperative course the patients (of this study) remain free from rejection in the further course.

• The individual HLA compatibility has no influence on the frequency of rejection.

The grade of compatibility in the HLA-DR locus seems to be associated with the different clinical features of rejection.

• The occurrence and the clinical symptomatology of hyperacute rejection is demonstrated in two patients of this study.

THE ESSENTIAL CLINICAL CONSEQUENCES OF THIS STUDY ARE AS FOLLOWS:

I. HISTOLOGICAL EXAMINATION

• Routine biopsies taken on a regular basis postoperatively can be reduced of are no longer necessary because findings only detectable by such routine histological examination do not require any treatment and are therefore without any clinical consequence.

• The relevance of the histological examination for a safe and exact diagnosis-making can be confirmed. However, the possibilities and results of the cytology should be especially considered in this respect. (See Chapter 2.)

II. HYPERACUTE REJECTION

• The existence of hyperacute rejection in liver transplantation could be demonstrated experimentally as well as clinically.

• Predisposing situations for hyperacute rejection still have to be analyzed in more detail in order to avoid such kinds of rejections.

• In case of an unexpected initial nonfunction or sudden unexplainable worsening of graft function in the early postoperative phase the possibility of a hyperacute rejection should be considered.

III. HLA COMPATIBILITY

• A consideration of the HLA compatibility for clinical donor-recipient-combinations of allocation is (still) not indicated at present.

• The relationship between HLA compatibility and different clinical features of rejection in conjunction with findings of other investigators indicate a clinical relevance of the histocompatibility in liver transplantation.

• This study was one of the reasons to stimulate the multicenter trial named L'ESPRIT and mentioned above.

REFERENCES

Adams DH, Burnett D, Stockley RA, McMaster P, Elias E (1987) Markers of biliary epithelial damage in liver allograft rejection. Transplant Proc 19: 3820-3821.

Adams DH, Neuberger JM (1990) Patterns of graft rejection following liver transplantation. J Hepatology 10: 113-119.

Ascher NL, Stock PG, Bumgardner GL, Payne WD, Najarian JS (1988) Infection and rejection of primary hepatic transplant in 93 consecutive patients treated with triple immunosuppressive therapy. Surg Gynecol Obstet 167: 474-484.

Behrend M, Steinhoff G, Wonigeit K, Pichlmayr R (1991) Patterns of adhesion molecule expression in human liver allografts. Transplant Proc 23: 1419-1420.

Binns RM (1967) Bone marrow and lymphoid cell injection of the pig foetus resulting in transplantation tolerance or immunity, and immunoglobulin production. Nature 214: 179-181.

Birtch AG, Orr WM, Duquella J (1968) Evaluation of horse anti-dog antilymphocyte globulin in the treatment of hepatic allografts. Surg Forum 19: 186-188.

Bockhorn H, Grotelüschen B, Tidow G, Lauchart W, Ziegler H, Coburg A, Schmidt E, Lesch P, Taegder K, Pfeiffer A, Seidler D, Trautwein G, Pichlmayr R (1972) Die allogene schweinelebertransplantation. eine funktionelle, enzymatische und morphologische Studie unter Berücksichtigung der Frage der Abstoßung oder immunologischen Toleranz. Langenbcek Arch Chir Suppl 135-138.

Bockhorn H, Lauchart W, Ringe B, Nedden H, Pichlmayr R (1975) SLA-Testung und MCL-Reaktion beim Schwein und ihre Beziehung zur Abstoßung von Haut- und Lebertransplantaten. Langenb Arch Chir Suppl 141-145.

Bornscheuer A, Gubernatis G, Ringe B, Lübbe N,

Grosse H, Schaps D, Kirchner E (1988) Ausbleibender anstieg des Sauerstoffverbrauchs nach Revaskularisierung der Leber: Ein sicheres Zeichen für eine initiale Nichtfunktion des transplantierten Organs? Z Gastroenterol 26: 10.

Bunke O (1959/60) Neue Konfidenzintervalle für den Parameter der Binomialverteilung. Wiss Zeitschr d. Humboldt-Universität Berlin 9: 335-363.

Calne RY, White HJO, Yoffa DE, Maginn RR, Binns RM, Samuel JR, Molina VP (1967a) Observations of orthotopic liver transplantation in the pig. Brit Med J 2: 478-480.

Calne RY, White HJO, Yoffa DE, Binns RM, Maginn RR, Herbertson RM, Millard PR, Molina VP, Davis DR (1967b) Prolonged survival of liver transplants in the pig. Brit Med J 4: 745-648.

Calne RY, White HJO, Binns RM, Herbertson BM, Millard PR, Pena J, Salaman JR, Samuel JR, Davis DR (1969a) Immunosuppressive effects of the orthotopically transplanted porcine liver. Transplant Proc 1: 321-324.

Calne RY, Sells RA, Penna JR, Davis DR, Millard PR, Hertertson BM, Binns RM, Danz DAL (1969b) Induction of immunologic tolerance by porcine liver allografts. nature 223: 472-476.

Calne RY, Williams R (1979) Liver transplantation. Cur probl Surg 16: 3-44.

Calne RY (1983a) Liver transplantation. Grune and Stratton, New York London Paris San Diego San Franzisko Sao Paulo Sydney Tokio Toronto.

Calne RY (1983b) Diagnosis of rejection. In: Roy Y. Calne (Hrsg.): Liver Transplantation: 199-200.

Calne RY (1991) Strategies in tolerance and liver transplantation Clin Transplantation 5: 544-548.

Colonna JO, Goldstein LI, Brems JJ, Vargas JH,

Brill JE, Berquist WJ, Hiatt JR, Busuttil RW (1987) A prospective study on the use of monoclonal anti-T3-cell antibody (OKT3) to treat steroid-resistant liver transplant rejection. Arch Surg 122: 1121-1123.

Daar AS, Fuggle SV, Fabre JW, Ting A, Morris PJ (1984) The detailed distribution of HLA-A,B,C antigens in normal human organs. Transplantation 38: 287-292.

Delmonico Fl, Cosimi AB (1988) Monoclonal antibody treatment of human allograft recipients. Surg, Gynecol Obstet 166: 89-98.

Demetris AJ, Lasky S, Van Thiel DH, Starzl TE, Dekker A (1985) Pathology of hepatic transplantation. Am J Pathol 118: 151-161.

Dent DM, Hickman R, Uys CJ, Saunders S, Terblanche J (1971) The natural history of liver allo- and autotransplantation in the pig. Brit J Surg 58: 407-413.

Donaldson PT, O'Grady J, Portman B, Davis H, Alexander GJM, Neuberger, Thick M, Calne RY, Williams R (1987) Evidence for an immune response to HLA class I antigens in the vanishing-bile duct syndrome after liver transplantation. Lancet 1: 945-948.

Egging HF, Hofstee N, Gips Ch, Krom RAF, Houthoff HJ (1984) Histopathology of serial graft biopsies from liver transplant recipients. Liver Homograft Pathology 114: 18-31.

Eid A, Moore SB, Wiesner Rh, Degoey SR, Nielson A, Krom RAF (1990) Evidence that the liver does not always protect the kidney from hyperacute rejection in combined liver-kidney transplantation across a positive lymphocyte crossmatch. Transplantation 50: 331-334.

Engemann R (1985) Die orthotope Lebertransplantation. Funktionelle, morphologische und immunologische Unterschungen zur Toleranz allogener Rattenlebertransplantate. Habilitationsschrift Medizinische Fakultät der Christian-Albrechts-Universität zu Kiel.

Esquivel CO, Jaffe R, Gordon RD, Iwatsuki S, Shaw Bw, Starzl TE (1985) Liver rejection and its differentiation from other causes of graft dysfunction. Sem Liver Dis 5: 369-374.

Fonkalsrud EW, Shafey OA, Ono H, Longmire WP (1966) Experience with orthotopic dog liver allografts. Surg Forum 17: 215-220.

Fonkalsrud EW, Ono H, Shafey OA, Longmire WP (1967) Orthotopic canine liver homo-

transplantation without vena cava interruption. Surg Gynecol Obstet 125: 319-327.

Forster PF, Sankary H, Williams JW (1988) Study of eosinophilia and hepatic dysfunction as a predictor of rejection in human liver transplantation. Transpl Proc 20: 676-677.

Fung JJ, Makowka L, Griffin M, Duquesnoy R, Tzakis A, Starzl TE (1987a) Successful sequential liver-kidney transplantation in patients with preformed lymphocytotoxic antibodies. Clin Transplant 1: 187-194.

Fung J, Griffin M, Duquesnoy R, Shaw B, Starzl TE (1987b) Successful sequential liver-kidney transplantation in a patient with preformed lymphocytotoxic antibodies. Transplant Proc 19: 767.

Garnier H, Clot JP, Chomette G (1970) Orthotopic transplantation of the porcine liver. Surg Gynecol Obstet: 105-111.

Georgii A, Wonigeit K, Worch KJ, Ringe B, Kemnitz J, Bunzendahl H, Helmke M, Pichlmayr R, Fennell RH (1986) Infection after orthotopic grafting of liver. Transplant Proc 18: 146-148.

Gordon RD, Fung JJ, Markus B, Fox I, Ivatsuki S, Esquivel CO, Tzakis A, Todo S, Starzl TE (1986) The antibody crossmatch in liver transplantation. Surgery 100: 705-715.

Grond S, Gouw ASH, Poppema S, Slooff MSH, Gips CH (1986) Chronic rejection in liver transplants: A histopathologic analysis of failed grafts and antecedent serial biopsies. Transplant Proc 18 Suppl 4: 128-135.

Groth CG, Porter KA, Otte JG, Daloze PM, Marchioro TL, Bretschneider L, Starzl TE (1968) Studies of blood flow and ultrastructural changes in rejecting and nonrejecting canine orthotopic liver homografts. Surgery 63, 658-668.

Gubernatis G, Lauchart W, Jonker M, Steinhoff G, Bornscheuer A, Neuhaus P, Van Es AA, Kemnitz J, Wonigeit K, Pichlmayr R (1987) Signs of hyperacute rejection of liver grafts in rhesus monkeys after donor-specific presensitization. Transplant Proc 19: 1082-1083.

Gubernatis G, Tusch G, Bornscheuer A, Raygrotzki S, Farle M, Kuse E, Bunzendahl H, Ringe B (1988a) Diagnose der initialen Nichtfunktion nach Lebertransplantation. Z Gastroenterol 26: 25-26.

Gubernatis G, Tusch G, Kuse E, Bornscheuer A,

Ringe B, Pichlmayr R (1988b) Ischämieschaden der Leber nach Transplantation: Symptomatologie und Differenzierung zwischen Reversibilität und Irreversivilität mit Hilfe eines Score. Langenbeck Arch Chir Suppl: 377-381.

Gubernatis G, Abendroth D, Haverich A, Bunzendahl H, Illner WD, Meyer HJ, Land W, Pichlmayr R (1988c) Technik der Mehrorganentnahme. Der Chirurg 59: 461-468.

Gubernatis G, Kemnitz J, Tusch G, Pichlmayr R (1988d) HLA compatibility and different features of liver allograft rejection. Transplant Int 1: 155-160.

Gubernatis G, Müller R, Riedel T, Pichlmayr R (1988e) HLA and liver allograft rejection: any influence? Eurotransplant Newsletter 59: 9.

Gubernatis G, Tusch G, Ringe B, Bunzendahl H, Pichlmayr R (1989a) Score-aided decision making in severe liver damage after hepatic transplantation. World J Surg 13: 259-265.

Gubernatis G, Bornscheuer A, Taki Y, Farle M, Lübbe N, Yamaoka Y, Beneking M, Burdelski M, Oellerich M (1989b) Total oxygen consumption, ketone body ratio and a special score are early indicators of irreversible liver allograft non-function. Transpl Proc 21: 2279-2281.

Gubernatis G, Kemnitz, J, Tusch G, Ringe B, Bunzendahl H, Riedel T, Müller R, Pichlmayr R (1989c) Different features of acute liver allograft rejection, their outcome and their possible relationship to HLA-compatibility. Transpl Proc 21: 2213-2214.

Gubernatis G, Kemnitz J, Bornscheuer A, Kuse E, Pichlmayr R (1989d) Potential various apperiances of hyperacute rejection in human liver transplantation. Langenbecks Arch Chir 374: 240-244.

Gubernatis G, Abendroth D, Haverich A, Bunzendahl H, Illner WD, Meyer HJ, Land W, Pichlmayr R (1989e) Multiple organ harvesting. Eurotransplant Newsletter 63: 6-19.

Gubernatis G (1989f) Techniques of organ procurement and preservation of liver and pancreas. Bailliere's Clinical Gastroenterology 3: 799-811.

Haverich A, Scott WC, Dawkins KD, Billingham ME, Jamieson SW (1984) Asymmetric pattern of rejection following orthotopic cardiac transplantation in primates. Heart Transplantation 3: 280-285.

Hesselink EJ, Klompmaker IJ, Pruim J, Van Schilfegaarde R, Slooff MJH (1989a) Hepatic artery thrombosis after orthotopic liver transplantation—A fatal complication or an asymptomatic event. Transpl Proc 21: 2462.

Hesselink EJ, Klompmaker IJ, Grond J, Gouw Ash, Van Schilfegaarde R, Slooff MJH (1989b) Hepatic artery thrombosis (HAT) after orthotopic transplantation (OLT)—The influence of technical factors and rejection episodes. Transplant Proc 21: 2468.

Hoffmann MW, Wonigeit K, Steinhoff G, Behrend M, Herzbeck H, Flad HD, Pichlmayr R (1991) Tumor necrosis factor alpha and interleukin-1 beta in rejecting human liver grafts. Transplant Proc 23 No 1: 1421-1423.

Houssin D, Gugenheim J, Bellon B, Gigou BM, Charra M, Crongneau S, Bismuth H (1985) Absence of hyperacute rejection of liver allografts in hypersensitized rats. Transplant Proc 17: 293-295.

Huebscher SG, Adams DH, Buckels JA, McMaster P, Neuberger J, Elias E (1989) Massive haemorrhagic necrosis of the liver after liver transplantation. J Clin Pathol 42 (4): 360-370.

Hunt AC (1967) Pathology of liver transplantation in the pig. In: Read: The Liver. Colston Papers 14 Butterworths, London, 337-349.

Huntley RT, Taylor PD, Iwasaki Y, Marchioro TL, Jeejeebhoy H, Porter KA, Starzl TE (1966) The use of antilymphocyte serum to prolonge dog homograft survival. Surg Forum 17: 230-233.

Iwatsuki S, Iwaki Y, Kano T, Klintmalm G, Koep LJ, Weil R, Starzl TE (1981) Successful liver transplantation from crossmatch-positive donors. Transplant Proc 13: 286-288.

Kamada N, Davies H, Roser B (1981) Reversal of transplantation immunity by liver grafting. Nature 292: 840-842.

Kamada N, Calne R (1983) A surgical experience with five hundred 30 liver transplants in the rat. Surgery 93: 64-69.

Kamada N (1985) The immunology of experimental liver transplantation in the rat. Immunology 55: 369.

Kemnitz J, Ringe B, Helmke M, Pichlmayr R, Burdelski M, Wonigeit K, Choritz H, Georgii A (1986) Klassifikation der Abstoßungsreaktion in Lebertransplantaten. Verh Dtsch Ges Pathol 70: 458.

Kemnitz J, Cohnert TR (1987) Diagnostic criteria for liver allograft rejection. Am J Surg Pathol 11: 737-738.

Kemnitz J, Ringe B, Cohnert TR, Gubernatis G, Helmke M, Choritz H, Georgii A (1989a) Bile duct injury as a part of diagnostic criteria for liver allograft rejection. Hum Pathol 20: 132-143.

Kemnitz J, Gubernatis G, Bunzendahl H, Ringe B, Pichlmayr R, Georgii A (1989b) Criteria for the histopathological classification of liver allograft rejection and their clinical relevance. Transplant Proc 21: 2208-2210.

Kemnitz J, Haverich A, Gubernatis G, Cohnert TR (1989c) Rapid identification of viral infections in liver, heart and kidney allograft biopsies by in situ hybridization. Am J Surg Pathol 13: 80-83.

Kemnitz J (1991) The histopathological classification of liver allograft rejection. In: R. Engemann, H. Hamelmann (Hrsg.): Experimental and Clinical Liver Transplantation. Excerpta Medica (Elsevier Sci. Publ. B.V.) Amsterdam-New York-Oxford 9-14.

Kemnitz J (1992) Diagnosis of rejection in biopsy material of cardiac allografts. Pabst Lengerich—Wien—Berlin.

Kirby RM, McMaster P, Clemens D, Hubscher SG, Angrisani L, Sealey M, Gunson BK, Salt PJ, Buckels JAC, Adams DH, Jurewicz WAJ, Jain AB, Elias E (1987) Orthotopic liver transplantation: postoperative complications and their management. Br J Surg 74: 3-11.

Klintmalm GB, Nery JR, Husberg BS, Gonwa TA, Tillery GW (1989) Rejection in liver transplantation. Hepatology 10: 978-985.

Klintmalm GB (1991) Rejection therapies Dig Dis Sci 36 (10): 1431-1433.

Knechtle S, Kolbeck PC, Psuchimoto S, Coundouriotis A, Sanfilippo F, Bollinger RR (1987a) Hepatic transplantation into sensitized recipients. Transplantation 43: 8-12.

Knechtle SJ, Kulbeck PC, Tsuchimoto S, Coundouriotis F, Sanfilippo F, Bollinger RR (1987b) Humoral rejection of rat hepatic transplants by passive transfer of serum.

Transpl Proc 19: 1072-1076.

Kubota K, Ericzon BG, Reinholt FP (1990) Diagnosis of liver transplant rejection by bile cytology Transplant Proc 22: 1521.

Kubota K, Ericzon BG, Barkholt L, Reinholt FP (1989) Bile cytology in orthotopic liver transplantation. Transplantation 48: 998.

Kukral JC, Riveron E, Weaver J, Nyman B, Vaitys S, Barret B, Starzl TE (1966) Metabolism of plasma protein fractions after orthotopic allografts and autografts of the canine liver. Surg Forum 17: 218-220.

Land W, Hillebrand G, Illner WD, Abendroth D, Hancke E, Schleibner S, Hammer C, Racenberg J (1988) First clinical experience with a new TCR/CD3-monoclonal antibody (BMA 031) in kidney transplant patients. Transplant Int 1: 116-117.

Land W (1991) Monoclonal antibodies in 1991: New potential options in clinical immunosuppressive therapy. Clin Transplant 5: 493-500.

Lauchart W (1986) Ergebnisse der Lebertransplantation bei erwachsenen Zirrhosepatienten. Analyse verschiedener Klassifikationen und prognostischer Faktoren. Habilitationsschrift Medizinische Hochschule Hannover.

Margreiter R, Kornberger R, Koller J, Steiner E, Spielberger M, Aigner F, Schmid T, Vogel W (1988) Can a liver graft from the same donor protect a kidney from rejection? Transplant Proc 20: 522-523.

Markus BH, Fung JJ, Gordon RD, Vanek M, Starzl TE, Duquesnoy RJ (1987) HLA histocompatibility and liver transplant survival. Transplant Proc 19: 63-65.

Maury CPJ, Teppo AM, Höckerstedt K (1988) Acute phase proteins and liver allograft rejection. Liver 8: 75-79.

McDonald JA, Painter DM, Bell R, Gallagher ND, Sheil AGR, McCaughan GW (1989) Human liver allograft rejection: Severity, prognosis, and response to treatment. Transplant Proc 21: 3792-3793.

Merion RM, Campbell DA, Dafoe DC, Rosenberg L, Turcotte JG, Juni JE (1988) Observations on quantitative scintigraphy with deconvolutional analysis in liver transplantation. Transplant Proc 20: 695-697.

Mikaeloff G, Rassat JP, Chabert M, Dumont L, Belleville J, Trouchon J, Malluret J, Descotes

J (1965) Transplantation orthotopique de foie chez le chien. Technique et résultats. Mem Acad Chir 91: 286-288.

Mikaeloff P, Pichlmayr R, Rassat JP, Messmer K, Bornel J, Tidow G, Etiennemartin M, Malluret J, Belleville P, Jonvenceau A, Falconnet J, Descotes J, Brendel W (1967) Homotransplantation orthotopique du foie chez le chien: Traitement immuno-dépresseur por sérum antilymphocyte. Presse Méd 75: 1967-1979.

Moore SB, Wiesner RH, Perkins JD, Nagorney DM, Sterioff S, Krom RAF (1987) A positive lymphocyte crossmatsch and majro histocompatibility complex mismatching do not predict early rejection of liver transplants in patients treated with cyclosporine. Transplant Proc 19: 2390-2391.

Mora NP, Klintmalm GB, Cofer JB et al (1990) Results after liver retransplantation (ReTx): A comparative study between "elective vs non-elective." ReTx. Transplant Proc 22 (4): 1509-1511.

Morel P, Rilo HLR, Tzakis AG, Todo S, Gordon RD, Starzl TE (1991) Liver retransplantation in adults: Overall results and determinant factors affecting the outcome. Transplant Proc 23 (6): 3029-3031.

Myburgh JA, Smit JA (1975) Prolongation of liver allograft survival by donor-specific soluble transplantation antigens and antigen-antibody complexes. Transplantation 19: 64-71.

Myburgh JA, Smit JA, Browde S, Hill RRH (1980) Transplantation tolerance in primates following lymphoid irradiation and allogeneic bone marrow injection. I. Orthotopic liver allografts. Transplantation 29: 401-404.

Neuberger J, Postmann B, Macdougall BRD, Calne RY, Williams R (1982) Recurrence of primary biliary cirrhosis after liver transplantation. N Engl J Med 306: 1-4.

Neuhaus P, Neuhaus R, Pichlmayr R, Vonnahme F (1982) An alternative technique of biliary reconstruction after liver transplantation. Res Exp Med 180: 239-245.

Oehlert W, Herfarth C, Zimmermann WE, Halbfass HJ, Hirschauer M, Körner H, Puff G, Schüfer H, Schneider N (1972) Das histologische Bild der transplantierten Schweineleber in seiner Beziehung zu Autoaggressionskrankheiten der Leber. Beitr Path 145, 37-50.

Oldhafer KJ, Gubernatis G, Tusch G, Kuse E, Pichlmayr R (1989) Gallesedimentcytologie: Eine neue, nichtinvasive Methode im postoperativen Monitoring nach Lebertransplantation. Langenbeck Arch Chir Suppl 421-425.

Oldhafer KJ, Gubernatis G, Ringe B, Pichlmayr R (1990) Experience with bile cytology after liver transplantation Transplant Proc 22: 1524.

Ozaki N, Ringe B, Bunzendahl H, Taki Y, Gubernatis G, Oellerich M, Kuse ER, Kiuchi T, Yamauchi K, Takada Y, Yamaguchi T, Ozawa K, Pichlmayr R (1991) Ketone body ratio as an indicator of early graft survival in clinical liver transplantation. Clin Transplant 5: 48-54.

Paintaud G, Miguet JP (1991) Diagnostic tools in liver allograft rejection J Hepatol 12: 256-260.

Peacock JH, Terblanche J (1967) Orthotopic homotransplantation of the liver in the pig. In: Read: The Liver. Colston Papers 14, Butterworth, London: 333-336.

Pichlmayr R, Brendel W, Mikaeloff P, Wiebecke B, Rassat JP, Pichlmayr I, Bomel J, Fateh-Moghadam A, Thierfelder S, Messmer K, Descotes J, Knedel M (1968) Survival of renal and liver homograft in dogs treated with heterologous antilymphocyte serum. In: Dausset, Hamburger, Mathe: Advances in transplantation, Munksgaard, Kopenhagen: 147-154.

Pichlmayr R, Brölsch Ch, Neuhaus P, Lauchart W, Grosse H, Creutzig H, Schnaidt U, Vonnahme F, Schmidt E, Burdelski M, Wonigeit K (1983) Report on 68 human orthotopic liver transplantations with special reference to rejection phenomena. Transplant Proc 15: 1279-1283.

Pichlmayr R, Ringe B, Lauchart W, Wonigeit K (1987a) Liver transplantation. Transplant Proc 19: 103-112.

Pichlmayr R, Gubernatis G (1987b) Rejection of the liver and review of current immunosuppressive protocols. Transplant Proc 19: 4367-4369.

Porter KA (1988) The pathology of rejection in human liver allografts. Transplant Proc 20: 483-485.

Ray RA, Lewin KJ, Colonna J, Goldstein LI,

Busuttil RW (1988) The role of liver biopsy in evaluating acute allograft dysfunction following liver transplantation: a clinical histologic correlation of 34 liver transplants. Human Pathology 19: 835-848.

Riddel AG, Terblanche J, Peacock JH, Tierris EJ, Hunt AC (1968) Experimental liver transplantation in pigs. In: Dausset, Hamburger, Mathe: Advances in Transplantation, 2. Aufl., Munksgaard, Kopenhagen: 639-641.

Roberti I, Lieberman KV, Manzarbeitia C, Schwartz M, Reisman L, Miller C (1992) Evidence that the systematic analysis of bile cytology permits monitoring of hepatic allograft rejection. Transplantation 54: 471-474.

Sankary HN, Williams JW, Foster PF (1988) Can serum liver function tests differentiate rejection from other causes of liver dysfunction after hepatic transplantation? Transplant Proc 20: 669-670.

Shaw BW, Gordon RD, Iwatsuki S, Starzl TE (1985a) Hepatic retransplantation. Transplant Proc 17: 264.

Shaw BW, Gordon RD, Iwatsuki S, Starzl TE (1985b) Retransplantation of the liver. Seminars in Liver Disease 5: 394.

Snover DC, Sibley RK, Freese DK (1984) Orthotopic liver transplantation: a pathological study of 63 serial liver biopsies from 17 patients with special reference to the diagnostic features and natural history of rejection. Hepatology 4: 1212-1222.

Snover DC (1986) The pathology of acute rejection. Transplant Proc 18: 123-127.

Snover DC, Freese DK, Sharp HL, Bloomer JR, Najarian JS, Ascher NL (1987) Liver allograft rejection: an analysis of the use of biopsy in determining outcome of rejection. Am J Surg Pathol 11: 1-10.

Snover DC (1989) Problems in the interpretation of liver biopsies after liver. transplantation Am J Surg Pathol 13 (1): 31-38.

Snover DC (1990) Liver transplantation In: G.E. Sale (Hrsg.): The pathology of organ transplantation. Butterworth (Boston-London-Singapur-Sydney-Toronto-Wellington) 103-132.

Starzl TE, Marchioro TL, Porter KA, Taylor PD, Faris TD, Herrmann TJ, Hlad CJ, Waddell WR (1965) Factors determining short- and long-term survival after orthotopic liver homotransplantation in the dog. Surgery 58:

131-155.

Starzl TE, Marchioro TL, Faris TD, Mccardle RJ, Iwasaki Y (1966) Avenues of future research in homotransplantation of the liver: With particular reference to hepatic supportive procedures, antilymphocyte serum and tissue typing. Am J Surg 112: 391-400.

Starzl TE (1969) Experience in hepatic transplantation. Saunders WB, Philadelphia: 164.

Starzl TE, Ishikawa M, Putnam CW, Porter KA, Picache R, Husberg BS, Halgrimson CG, Schroter G (1974) Progress in and deterrents to orthotopic liver transplantation, with special reference to survival, resistance to hyperacute rejction, and biliary duct reconstruction. Transplant Proc 6: 129-139.

Starzl TE, Iwatsuki S, Shaw BW, Gordon RD, Esquivel CO (1985) Immunosuppression and other nonsurgical factors in the improved results of liver transplantation. Sem Liver Dis 5: 334.

Starzl TE, Demetris AJ, Todo S, Kang YG, Tzakis A, Duquesnoy R, Makowka L, Banner B, Concepcion W, Porter KA (1989) Evidence of hyperacute rejection of human liver grafts: The case of the canary kidneys. Clin Transplant 3: 37-45.

Steinhoff G, Wonigeit K, Pichlmayr R (1988a) Analysis of sequential changes in major histocompatibility complex expression in human liver grafts after transplantation. Transplantation 45: 394-401.

Steinhoff G, Wonigeit K, Pichlmayr R (1988b) Polymorphic HLA-A and HLA-B antigens are induced in rejecting liver grafts. Transplant Proc 20: 698-700.

Steinhoff G, Jonker M, Gubernatis G, Wonigeit K, Lauchart W, Bornscheuer A, Nashan B, Pichlmayr R (1990a) The course of untreated acute rejection and effect of repeated anti-CD3 monoclonal antibody treatment in rhesus monkey liver transplantation. Transplantation 49: 669-674.

Steinhoff G, Behrend M, Pichlmayr R (1990b) Induction of ICAM-1 on hepatocyte membranes during liver allograft rejection and infection. Transplant Proc 22 (5): 2308-2309.

Steinhoff G (1990c) Major histocompatibility complex antigens in human liver transplants. J Hepatol 11: 9-15.

Steiniger B, Klempnauer J, Wonigeit K (1984)

Phenotype and histological distribution of interstitial dendritic cells in the rat pancreas, liver, heart and kidney. Transplantation 38: 169-175.

Struck E, Nitschke J, Laus J, Schaltenberg PJ, Hamelmann H (1977) Orthotope Lebertransplantation. Die Vorbereitung ihrer klinischen Anwendung. Witzstrock, Baden-Baden-Köln-New York.

Stuart FP, Torres E, Hester WJ, Dammin GJ, Moore FD (1967) Orthotopic autotransplantation and allotransplantation of the liver: Functional and structural patterns in the dog. Ann Surg 165: 325-340.

Takada Y, Ozaki N, Ringe B, Mori K, Gubernatis G, Oellerich M, Yamaguchi T, Kiuchi T, Shimahara Y, Yamaoka Y, Sakurai K, Ozawa K, Pichlmayr R (1992) Receiver operating characteristic (ROC) analysis of the ability of arterial ketone body ratio to predict graft outcome after liver transplantation—its sensitivity and specificity. Transplant Int 5: 23-26.

Taki Y, Gubernatis G, Yamaoka Y, Oellerich M, Yamamoto Y, Ringe B, Ikamoto R, Bunzendahl H, Beneking M, Burdelski M, Bornscheuer A, Ozawa K, Pichlmayr R (1990) Significance of arterial ketone body ratio measurement in human liver transplantation. Transplantation 49: 535-539.

Terblanche J, Peacock JH, Bowes J, Davies RP, Tierris EJ, Palmer DB, Hunt AC (1967) The use of the pig as an experimental animal for orthotopic liver homotransplantation. Brit J Surg 54: 231.

Thorogood J. For the L'ESPRIT group: Relationship between HLA compatibility and first liver allograft survival. Transplant Proc (in press).

Tzakis AG (1985) The dearterialized liver graft. Sem Liver Dis 5: 375-376.

Vierling JM, Fennell RH (1985) Histopathology of early and late human hepatic allograft rejection: evidence of progressive destruction of interlobular bile ducts. Hepatology 5: 1076-1082.

Weber E (1980) Grundriß der biologischen Statistik 8. Auflage, Fischer, Stuttgart New York.

Westra Al, Romaniuk A, Ryffa T, Wildevuur CH, Nieuwenhuis P (1987) Infiltration pattern of rat heart allografts during rejection. Transplant Proc 19: 374.

Wight DGD (1983a) Pathology of rejection. In: Roy Y. Calne (Hrsg.): Liver Transplantation. 247-277.

Wight DGD (1983b) Pathology of liver transplantation (other than rejection) In: Roy Y. Calne (Hrsg.): Liver Transplantation: 289-316.

Whight L, Manez R, Kusne S, Martin M, Demetris J, Starzl TE, Duquesnoy R (in press) Association between donor-recipient HLA-DR compatibility and cytomegalovirus (CMV) hepatitis and chronic rejection in liver transplantation. Transplant Proc.

Wood RP, Shaw BW, Williams L (1988) The use of OKT3 rescue therapy after orthotopic liver transplantation—The University of Nebraska Medical Center Experience. Transplant Proc 20: 254-259.

Yates Y (1980) In: E. Weber (Hrsg.) Grundriß der biologischen Statistik 8. Auflage, Fischer, Stuttgart New York.

Zimmermann FA, Davies HS, Knoll PP, Gokel JM, Schmidt T (1984) Orthotopic liver allografts in the rat. The influence of strain combinations on the fate of the graft. Transplantation 37, 406-410.

CHAPTER 2

TRANSPLANT ASPIRATION CYTOLOGY OF THE LIVER

Hans Jürgen Schlitt, Björn Nashan

INTRODUCTION

After liver transplantation various pathologic conditions can lead to graft dysfunction. Among these conditions, differentiation of acute rejection from nonimmunologic causes of graft damage is of particular relevance because of the completely different therapeutic approaches. Although a number of noninvasive methods can help to differentiate the causes of graft dysfunction, the most reliable method is the evaluation of morphological changes in a representative specimen of organ tissue, usually obtained by a biopsy. Histology of such tissue specimens is the established method for morphological evaluation of intragraft processes, and histologic findings for different pathologic entities in liver grafts have been well defined (Snover et al 1987, Wight et al 1987, Ludwig 1988, Portmann et al 1987). However, transcutaneous core biopsies of liver grafts carry a certain risk of bleeding complications, particularly in patients with severe graft dysfunction with markedly reduced plasma coagulation factors and low thrombocyte counts, and require a workup time of several hours. Such biopsies are usually performed only with clinical indications, i.e., in case of liver dysfunction, or as protocol biopsies for study purposes at longer intervals.

In contrast, aspiration biopsies performed by very thin needles are a very safe procedure for obtaining graft specimens for morphologic evaluation. This method was introduced for evaluation of kidney allografts by the Helsinki group more than 20 years ago (Pasternack et al 1973) and has since been developed into a clinically useful procedure (Häyry et al 1981, von Willebrand et al 1984). The Innsbruck group was the first to apply this method to liver grafts (Vogel et al 1984) and subsequently several centers have used it for evaluation of intragraft events in liver-transplanted patients (Lautenschlager et al 1988a, Fehrman et al 1988, Greene et al 1988a, Kirby et al 1988, Schlitt et al 1989, Nashan et al 1989, Carbonnel et al 1990, Schlitt et al 1991a, Kubota et al 1991, Lautenschlager et al 1991a) and have analyzed its potency in animal models (Lautenschlager et al 1988b). Because of the more complex pathologic processes after liver transplantation as compared to kidney transplantation, graft cytology of the liver did not unanimously receive credit at the outset. With growing experience, however, the method has become a routine procedure for monitoring liver allografts in several transplant centers. Although the informative value of the method is restricted to certain questions, in experienced hands it can provide important information on the state of the graft and particularly on immunological processes occurring in the graft. Thus, aspiration cytology can be very helpful for the clinical management of liver grafted patients.

THE METHOD AND ITS EVALUATION

Performing aspiration biopsies of liver grafts for cytologic evaluation requires very few materials, including a 25G spinal needle and 10 ml of a sterile cell culture medium containing antibiotics, heparin, and human albumin (Fig. 1). Localization of the optimal biopsy site by bedside ultrasound examination is usually not necessary but may be helpful in special situations, e.g. after transplantation of a small or segmental graft into a large abdominal cavity where interposition of bowel between the abdominal wall and the graft may occur. The standard and optimal biopsy site is anterolaterally into the right lobe of the liver; alternatively, a right subcostal biopsy into liver segment IV is also possible and sometimes more convenient for the patient. Because of the short duration of the procedure and the small diameter of the biopsy needles used, local anesthesia is not required and the biopsy is well tolerated by the patients. After more than 3,000 aspiration biopsies, some of which have been performed in patients with severe coagulopathy and thrombocytopenia, no complications due to the procedure have been observed (Schlitt et al 1993a). Thus, aspiration biopsies can be safely performed in any clinical situation. Due to the use of very thin needles even an accidental puncture of the bowel—which is usually discovered by the microscopic findings in the aspirate—remains without clinical relevance and does not require any specific therapy.

At the time of the biopsy one or two drops of venous blood are obtained and diluted in

about 5 ml of the above mentioned culture medium for comparative reasons; both samples, aspirate and blood, are then analyzed in parallel. Aspirate and blood dilutions are cytocentrifuged onto glass slides at a density such that the erythrocytes just touch each other. Although more dense preparations would yield higher numbers of lymphocytes and hepatocytes per slide, it is not possible to evaluate the morphology of the mononuclear cells sufficiently under these conditions due to the horizontal compression of the cytoplasm of the cells. For routine staining a Romanowsky-Giemsa stain is used (Greene et al 1988b, Schlitt et al 1991a). If the aspirate is found to be representative, i.e., when at least 25 to 30 hepatocytes are present per slide, the aspirate and blood specimens are evaluated for the presence of immune activation, i.e., the presence of activated lymphocytes or blasts. In addition, the hepatocytes present in the aspirate are evaluated for their size and for cytoplasmic changes as well as for the extent and localization of bile pigment.

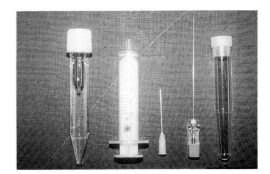

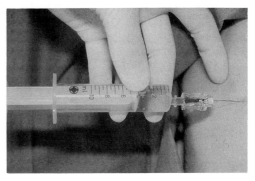

Fig. 1. Technical prerequisites for liver transplant aspiration cytology. (A) Material required: 25G spinal needle, other needle, culture medium, syringe, empty tube. (B) Performance of aspiration biopsy with graft aspirate visible in the cone of the needle.

While for aspiration biopsies of kidney grafts the calculation of a "total corrected increment" (Häyry et al 1981, von Willebrand et al 1984) as an indicator of the overall extent of intragraft immune activation has proved to be adequate, we prefer to use a more detailed description of the extent and pattern of immune activation in graft and blood and of the parenchymal changes. Due to the more complex pathophysiologic and immunologic changes that occur in liver grafts, this descriptive method seems to be better for differentiating the potential causes of graft dysfunction. For documentation purposes a semiquantitative scoring system is additionally applied to describe the extent of immune activation in aspirate (A 0-5) and blood (B 0-5), the morphology of hepatocytes (H 1-4) and the extent and localization of cholestasis (C 0-3, i (= intracellular) or e (= extracellular)); this scoring system has been previously described in more detail (Schlitt et al 1989, Schlitt et al 1991a) (Table 1). It must be noted, however, that the total corrected increment method has also been

described to be helpful for the evaluation of liver transplant aspiration cytology (TAC) (Lautenschlager et al 1988a)

Since preparation of the slides can be accomplished in about 20 minutes, the biopsy result can be available within half an hour after the biopsy has been taken. This is in marked contrast to the processing of a core biopsy which takes about four hours even when a rapid embedding procedure is used. Particularly in case of suspected rejection this allows a rapid clinical decision about the adequate treatment.

ACUTE LIVER GRAFT REJECTION IN ASPIRATION CYTOLOGY

Because of the unique ability of the method to reveal intragraft immune events in detail, aspiration cytology has proved to be particularly useful for the diagnosis or exclusion of acute cellular liver graft rejection.

In acute rejection, the typical finding is the presence of 20 to 50% of activated lymphocytes in the graft aspirate while no or only few activated cells are present in the blood (Schlitt et al 1991a). These activated lymphocytes are characterized by enlarged and more or less round nuclei with or without a condensed chromatin pattern and by an enlarged and basophilic cytoplasm (Fig. 2). Lymphoblasts which are characterized by even larger nuclei with one or more nucleoli inside may also be present in the graft during rejection but are usually not the predominant cell type, although the amount of blasts that appear during rejection may depend on the immunosuppressive protocol used (Lautenschlager et al 1988a, Schlitt et al 1992a). In severe rejection even mitotic figures of lymphocytes can be observed (Fig. 2). Parenchymal changes and the extent of cholestasis in acute rejection are highly variable and are, thus, of no diagnostic value. At the beginning of acute rejection eosinophilia is frequently detectable in aspirate and blood which is probably due to IL-5 production (Lautenschlager et al 1990). This eosinophilia, however, has not been shown to have an independent diagnostic relevance.

When scoring systems are applied to describe the immune activation, activation in the aspirate (A) is generally ≥2 with a considerable difference between activation in aspirate and in blood (A minus B ≤1.5) (Schlitt et al 1991a)

Table 1. Semiquantitative scoring of liver transplant aspiration cytology (TAC)

Scoring Parameters:
A	Immune Activation in Aspirate
B	Immune Activation in Blood
H	Hepatocyte Morphology
C	Extent of Cholestasis

Scoring:
A/B	0	No immune activation	
	1	< 10 %	of lymphocytes activated
	2	10-25 %	of lymphocytes activated
	3	25-50 %	of lymphocytes activated
	4	50-90 %	of lymphocytes activated
	5	> 90 %	of lymphocytes activated
	a	lymphocytes >30% of leukocytes	
	b	lymphocytes < 8% of leukocytes	

H	1	normal hepatocytes
	2	hepatocyte swelling/edema
	3	vacuolization
	4	necrosis

C	0	no cholestasis
	1	slight cholestasis
	2	moderate cholestasis
	3	severe cholestasis
	i	only intracellular
	e	mainly extracellular

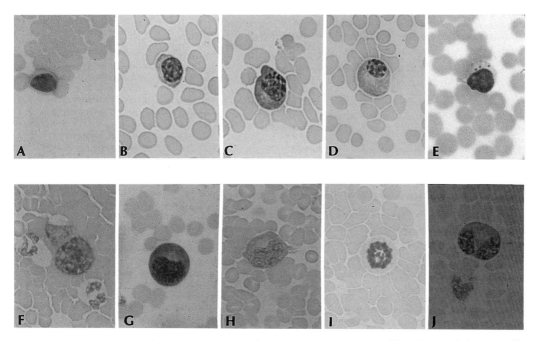

Fig. 2. Immune activation in liver TAC; Romanowsky-Giemsa staining: Normal lymphocyte (A), Minimally activated lymphocyte (B), Activated lymphocyte (C), Plasma cell (D), Large granular lymphocyte (E), Highly activated lymphocyte (F) Besides normal lymphocyte and two polymorphonuclear granulocytes, Lymphoblast (G), Monoblast (H), Early mitosis (I), Late mitosis (J) Besides normal lymphocyte.

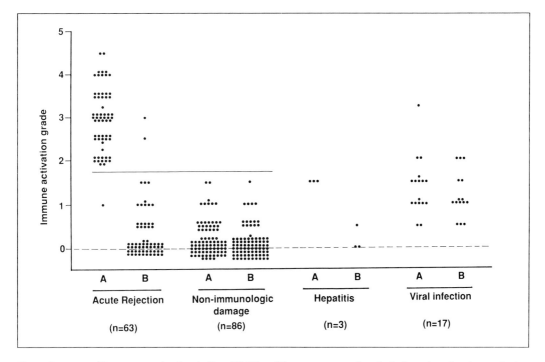

Fig. 3. Patterns of immune activation in liver TAC for different causes of graft dysfunction. Semiquantitative scoring (0-5) of immune activation in liver graft aspirate (A) and blood (B) was analyzed, showing clearly different patterns for acute rejection and nonimmunologic graft damage, and also typical patterns in hepatitis and systemic viral infection. (from: Schlitt HJ et al Transplantation 51:786, 1991a)

(Fig. 3). With the total corrected increment (TCI) method, a score of ≥3.5 is usually found in acute rejection (Lautenschlager et al 1991).

Evaluating the clinical reliability of the method, we found a high sensitivity for diagnosis of acute rejection (98.7% for the first two postoperative weeks) when cytologic results were retrospectively compared with the clinical course of the patients and—where available—with histologic findings. However, the specificity of the method proved to be rather low (76.5% for the first two postoperative weeks). Further analysis of these findings revealed that the negative predictive value was close to 100% while the positive predictive value was only around 50% (Nashan et al 1989, Schlitt et al 1991b, Schlitt et al 1992a). This means that in the absence of rejection-like immune activation in liver TAC acute graft rejection can be safely excluded. In contrast, however, the presence of rejection-like immune activation does not necessarily imply the presence of clinical rejection. At first view this result seemed to be disappointing, but analysis of histologic results of routinely performed core biopsies revealed a similarly

low positive predictive value (Schlitt et al 1992a, Snover et al 1987). Thus, both morphologic methods are obviously able to detect spontaneously reversible episodes of subclinical rejection (see below) and both are, unfortunately, not able to differentiate such episodes from clinically overt rejection which requires aggressive treatment. Other studies have found worse correlations between cytological and histological findings (Kirby et al 1988, Kubota et al 1991), but these studies relied on the total corrected increment method, did not specify the representativity of the analyzed biopsies and did not evaluate the clinical findings in the patients in detail.

A number of immunocytological stainings of TACs from rejecting livers have been performed (see below), but according to our experience and to all published data these stainings do not give additional diagnostic information for clinical practice.

The findings show that rejection-like immune activation in aspiration cytology can be regarded as necessary but not as sufficient for making the diagnosis of acute rejection. Thus, the cytologist detecting typical immune

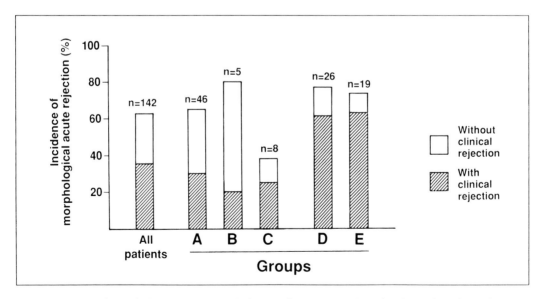

Fig. 4. Incidence of morphological acute cellular liver graft rejection with and without clinical manifestation for different immunosuppressive protocols. Patients in group A, D and E received quadruple drug therapy consisting of ATG, azathioprine, low dose steroids, and about 2 mg/kg/day cyclosporin starting either very early (d 0-1, group A), delayed (d 2-4, group D) or late (> d 4, group E) after transplantation, respectively. Patients in group B received quadruple therapy with early cyclosporin at 2 mg/kg/day, but with the monoclonal antibody BMA031 instead of ATG. Patients in group C were treated with 5 mg/kg/day cyclosporin from day 0 and low dose steroids only. (from: Schlitt HJ et al Transplantation 54:273, 1992a)

activation in the aspirate—even if it is very strong—must not make the diagnosis "acute rejection" and should only describe the presence of "immune activation consistent with acute rejection". Adequate interpretation of the result therefore requires close communication and co-operation between the cytologist and the physicians taking care of the patient.

OTHER CYTOLOGIC FINDINGS AND THEIR RELATION TO LIVER GRAFT DYSFUNCTION

Although the main focus of liver TAC is on the analysis of acute rejection, careful evaluation of the biopsy can reveal other patterns of immune activation and details of parenchymal changes and cholestasis. Thus, liver TAC can also provide evidence for liver dysfunction causes other than acute rejection (Schlitt et al 1991b, Lautenschlager et al 1991, Kubota et al 1991) (Figs. 2 and 5, Table 2).

Apart from acute clinical and subclinical rejection immune activation of mild to moderate degree can also be found in cases of *systemic viral infection*, particularly cytomegalovirus infection. In this situation, immune activation — sometimes even with some blasts—is present in

aspirate and in blood, although immune activation in the graft may be slightly stronger. Moreover, the number of small, i.e., nonactivated, lymphocytes is frequently increased and, in addition, lymphocytes carrying eosinophilic granules in their cytoplasm, so-called large granular lymphocytes (LGL), are frequently detectable (Lautenschlager et al 1990, Nashan et al 1991). Due to the presence of immune activation also in blood, the corrected increment is generally <5. In semiquantitative scoring there are usually findings that are described by A1a to A2a and B0-1 to B1-2.

In the few cases of *graft hepatitis* (mostly recurrent B hepatitis) which have been analyzed by aspiration cytology an increased amount of small lymphocytes, sometimes with very slight activation, i.e., enlarged cytoplasm without other signs of activation, and individual large granular lymphocytes were seen in the aspirate; the blood sample was normal in these patients (Schlitt et al 1991b).

Some—and in few cases even considerable—immune activation in aspirate and blood can also be observed in patients with *severe bacterial or fungal infections*. In contrast to acute rejection, immune activation in these cases is predomi-

Table 2. Most frequent TAC findings and their diagnostic relevance

TAC Finding	Diagnostic Relevance
Immune activation in aspirate >> blood (mainly activated lymphocytes)	Acute rejection possible
Slight immune activation in aspirate and blood (mainly activated lymphocytes and LGLs)	Suggestive of viral infection
Slight immune activation in aspirate and blood (mainly blasts)	Suggestive of parainfectious immune activation
Hepatocyte swelling	Very frequent finding without pathological relevance
Vacuolization of hepatocytes	First 4-5 days: normal finding Thereafter: evidence for more severe parenchymal damage
Intracellular cholestasis	Sign of parenchymal damage
Extracellular cholestasis	First 4-5 days: normal finding Thereafter: suggestive of biliary obstruction or cholangitis

nated by blastoid cells. Their presence is probably due to a nonspecific activation of mononuclear cells by lymphokines released during the infectious process. In rare cases when such cells are preferentially present in the aspirate it may be difficult to decide whether this is still due to infection or whether it reflects an incipient rejection. In this case probably daily monitoring by TAC, performance of a core biopsy,

and intensive discussions between cytologist and clinician are particularly important for deciding about the adequate therapeutic strategy.

Parenchymal damage of variable extent is frequently found in the aspiration biopsies. Even in uneventful courses after liver transplantation the hepatocytes are markedly swollen during the first four to five postoperative days in most cases. Afterwards, these morphologic changes

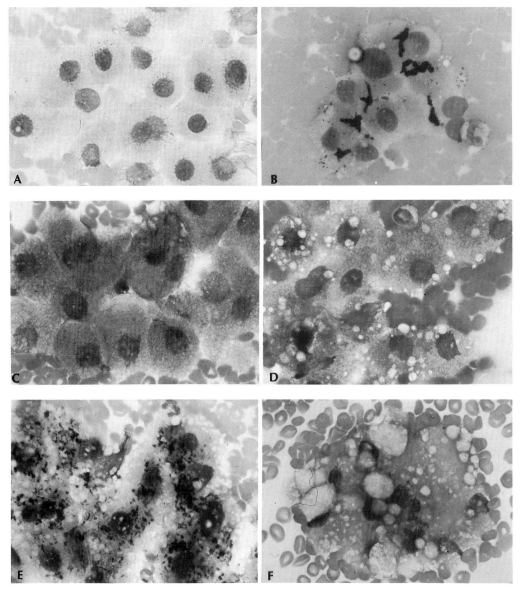

Fig. 5. Parenchymal changes in liver TAC; Romanowsky-Giemsa staining: Normal hepatocytes (A), Normal hepatocytes with extracellular cholestasis (B), Swollen hepatocytes (C), Swollen hepatocytes with isometric vacuolization (D), Swollen hepatocytes with isometric vacuolization and marked intracellular cholestasis (E), Hepatocytes with anisometric vacuolization (fatty degeneration) (F).

normalize slowly and completely normal hepatocytes are usually not seen before the third or fourth postoperative week. Even vacuolization of the hepatocytes is not uncommon in the first week, but it quickly disappears over a few days unless *severe preservation/reperfusion damage* has occurred; in this case vacuolization may even deteriorate from day to day and intracellular cholestasis will then increase rapidly.

The presence of mild to moderate extracellular cholestasis in the first postoperative week is also not unusual. The cause of this extracellular accumulation of bile even in liver grafts with very good early function is not clear; it can only be speculated that it might be caused by an obstruction of small bile canaliculi by the postoperative edema of the hepatocytes. Only if early extracellular cholestasis is severe or if it persists for more than one week does it indicate a more central biliary obstruction. Similarly, extracellular cholestasis appearing later in the course can be an indicator of *biliary obstruction or cholangitis* and should lead to the performance of additional diagnostic procedures for verifying or abandoning these diagnoses.

Swollen hepatocytes with extensive isometric vacuolization and intracellular accumulation of bile pigment are a nonspecific indicator of major parenchymal damage. In most cases, these changes reflect either ischemic graft damage due to general hemodynamic problems or vascular complications, or severe *preservation/reperfusion injury*, particularly if they are present from the beginning. Although quantitation of the damage by cytology is not possible, the presence of normal or only mildly altered hepatocytes on the same slide indicates a more focal (usually pericentral) damage which has a better prognosis than diffuse parenchymal injury. In contrast, detection of large anisometric vacuoles in hepatocytes that are otherwise normal and that have no or only very mild cholestasis is more specific and usually indicates *fatty degeneration* of the liver, the vacuoles representing fat accumulations in the liver cells.

Macrophages are usually very rare in graft aspirates but their number can increase remarkably in certain situations. Macrophages are large cells with cytoplasmic vacuoles which can contain a variety of materials from cellular debris to bile pigment. Due to their extensive phagocytic activity they tend to have a huge cytoplasm and a compressed, frequently bone-shaped nucleus of monocyte-like structure. The presence of these cells demonstrates that major parenchymal damage to the graft has occurred which is now repaired. However, this finding is also nonspecific and the extent of macrophage infiltration has no independent prognostic value (Lautenschlager et al 1988a, Vogel et al 1984) (Fig. 6).

Remarkably, in some patients red cell precursors like normoblasts and erythroblasts can be observed in the aspirate. The origin and the relevance of these cells in the graft is not clear, but their condensed chromatin pattern (normoblasts) and their large blastoid nuclei and basophilic cytoplasm (basophilic erythroblasts) may lead to a confusion with activated lymphocytes and lymphoblasts.

The presence of pycnotic granulocytes or granulocyte clusters in the aspirate, particularly if large numbers of such cells are present, may indicate abscess formation in the liver or somewhere else along the path of the biopsy needle, e.g. a subphrenic abscess, infected ascites or intrapleural empyema (own unpublished observation). Therefore, such a finding should lead to additional diagnostic procedures by ultrasound or by a CT scan.

Turquoise-colored hemosiderin accumulations in hepatocytes are frequently observed and may be increased by perioperative transfusions administered to the graft recipient. They have no known pathological relevance. Bile duct epithelial cells are only rarely detected (Fig. 6).

DIAGNOSTIC LIMITS AND PROBLEMS OF THE METHOD

As a cytological method liver TAC has a number of advantages, the most prominent of which is the possibility for detailed analysis of the mononuclear cells and their activation state. However, the method has certain clear limits concerning the evaluation of intragraft events and pathologic changes and, moreover, technical problems can interfere with adequate interpretation of the results (Table 3).

The most important prerequisite for obtaining reliable results is that the biopsy really reflects the intragraft compartment and does

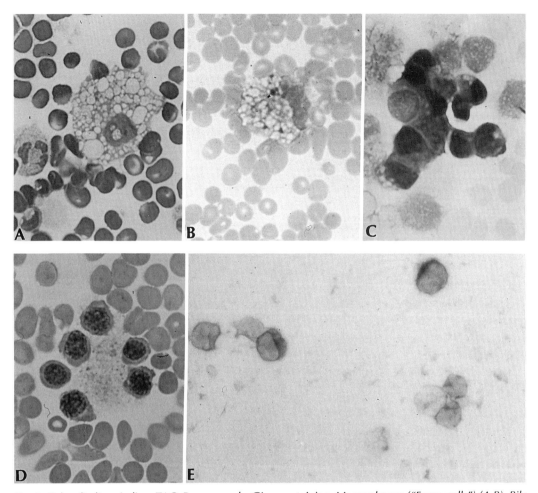

Fig. 6. *Other findings in liver TAC; Romanowsky-Giemsa staining: Macrophages ("Foam cells") (A,B), Bile duct epithelial cells (C), Red cell precursors (D), Donor lymphocytes (blue: donor HLA class I; brown: CD3⁺ T cells) (E).*

Table 3. Advantages and disadvantages of liver TAC

Advantages	Disadvantages
Detailed analysis of infiltrates (cell types, activation state)	No information about bile duct lesions and vascular changes
Some judgment of parenchymal damage	No information about cellular architecture (localization of infiltrates) and chronic changes
Safe method, applicable in any clinical situation	Interpretation sometimes impossible (blood, ascites)
Frequent monitoring easily possible	Interpretation of single biopsy sometimes difficult
Good acceptance by patients	
Rapid availability of results	

not only contain blood cells due to the accidental puncture of an intrahepatic blood vessel, i.e., the biopsy must be representative. To guarantee that, the—principally very easy—biopsy technique has to be standardized in a way that a sufficient quality of the aspirate is regularly achieved. Aspiration of a "bloody" biopsy cannot be avoided in all cases, but then it should be repeated immediately. An aspirate considered to be representative should contain at least 25-30 hepatocytes per slide even when the slide was prepared at a cell density in which the erythrocyte layer on the slide is not completely closed. A certain amount of (probably sinusoidal) blood is always present in the aspirate reflecting that the liver is as well vascularized organ. When smaller numbers of hepatocytes are present, however, it is very likely that the aspirate is severely spoiled by blood; such biopsies should not be evaluated. Similarly, evaluation of particularly dry biopsies, i.e., biopsies in which large numbers of hepatocytes but only very few erythrocytes are present, can be difficult. In this case blood contamination is almost completely absent and thus the intraparenchymal compartment of cells is overrepresented compared to a "standard" TAC. Since intrahepatic but extravascular cells are predominantly lymphocytes, the presence of considerable amounts of lymphocytes and only few granulocytes is the typical finding in dry biopsies. In most cases these dry biopsies can be evaluated, but overrepresentation of the parenchymal compartment has to be taken into account when interpreting the findings.

Concerning the evaluation of parenchymal abnormalities in the graft, aspiration cytology is, of course, of limited value. The relatively small number of hepatocytes gives a general impression about the presence or absence of gross parenchymal damage and may even give some hints regarding a potential underlying cause of damage in some cases. The localization of cellular infiltrations, bile duct morphology, and blood vessel changes, however, cannot be evaluated by aspiration cytology at all. Similarly, a quantitation and localization of parenchymal damage is not possible cytologically. A clear analysis of parenchymal changes, therefore, always requires histologic evaluation of a core biopsy. Thus, analysis of "rejection" by aspiration cytology always refers to "acute cellular rejection", the detection or exclusion of "chronic rejection" is completely beyond the abilities of this method.

As mentioned above, aspiration cytology is highly sensitive for detecting and analyzing intragraft immune events. However, it must be kept in mind that it only can describe morphological changes which do not necessarily correlate with the in vivo functional relevance of these changes. The obviously low specificity of liver TAC for diagnosing acute rejection is also shared by the histology and reflects the shortcomings of any morphological method (Schlitt et al 1992a). Thus, much care must be taken in interpreting cytologic findings to achieve a clinical diagnosis. Moreover, immune activation patterns and their clinical relevance are markedly influenced by the immunosuppressive regimens applied (Schlitt et al 1992a, Schlitt et al 1992b), again requiring caution in interpretation of the results, particularly when morphological and clinical findings obtained in different transplantation centers with different immunosuppressive regimens are compared.

Moreover, a very limited experience with liver TAC in pediatric patients suggests that acute rejection in these patients may also present with considerable immune activation in peripheral blood which is very rarely seen during rejection in adult patients. This demonstrates that TAC results in pediatric patients have to be interpreted with particular care. In addition, also in adult patients there may be cytologic findings of mixed and atypical patterns which may hamper straightforward interpretation. In this situation, the diagnostic potency may be increased by comparison with previous biopsy findings, particularly if they have been obtained at close intervals. However, core biopsies are required in many of these situations.

For a sensible application of liver TAC in clinical practice one must always be aware of the advantages, disadvantages, and problems of the method and must respect its diagnostic limits. Over interpretation of the results would rapidly lead to clinical disappointments and would then unduly discredit the method.

CLINICAL RELEVANCE OF CYTOLOGIC ROUTINE MONITORING

Close monitoring of liver grafted patients in order to get information about potentially dangerous changes as early as possible is highly important. Usually, such routine monitoring includes a variety of noninvasive tests like the analysis of blood biochemistry, daily evaluation of bile amount and color and, increasingly, frequent duplex ultrasonography. Immunologic monitoring by analysis of cell surface markers and subpopulations of peripheral blood mononuclear cells has been evaluated extensively, but has not proved to be of much clinical relevance so far. Thus, for a more effective immunologic monitoring information about the events in the graft itself are obviously required. Because of the small but clear risks of core biopsies, this method is not suitable for that purpose in clinical practice. Aspiration cytology, however, which is well tolerated by the patients, which carries almost no risk of complications, and which can be analyzed very quickly represents an ideal method for such monitoring (Schlitt et al 1993a).

With this method for monitoring of intragraft events at hand the question still remains about the clinical value of such an approach. To decide about this, several aspects must be considered: On the one hand, it was demonstrated that rejection-like immune activation without clinical signs of rejection ("subclinical rejection") is rather frequently observed but does not require specific treatment. This inability of the method to differentiate clinical from subclinical rejection indicates that a preclinical diagnosis of an acute rejection which may require treatment in the future is not possible. Therefore, the performance of routine biopsies for detecting episodes of "subclinical rejection" seems to be of no practical value. On the other hand, however, it could be shown that interpretation of cytologic findings in the aspirate is facilitated by evaluation of their changes over time. The presence of slight intragraft immune activation in a certain biopsy, for example, can be interpreted much better in the context of multiple biopsy results obtained at close intervals. With this additional information even complex cytologic patterns in an individual biopsy may be understood so that appropriate clinical consequences can be drawn or additional diagnostic procedures can be initiated (Greene et al 1988c, Nashan et al 1990). Moreover, with frequent monitoring the clinician has continuous information about the immunologic state of the graft so that in case of sudden graft dysfunction an "emergency" biopsy in the night or on weekends may become unnecessary in many cases.

In addition, in patients with severe infectious complications routine monitoring can be helpful for the management of immunosuppressive therapy. If immune activation is completely absent, the immunosuppressive medication in such a patient can be reduced or even stopped without a particularly high risk of rejection. Frequent monitoring in the further course then helps to determine the necessity of reintroducing or increasing immunosuppressive treatment again. As long as immune activation is continuously absent immunosuppressive therapy can probably be withheld or kept at a low level, but as soon as immune activation reappears it should be increased or reintroduced (Fig. 7). Even if the reappearance of immune activation is associated with signs of graft dysfunction, thus indicating the presence of acute rejection, reintroduction of basic immunosuppression is often sufficient to normalize liver function in this high risk group of patients.

Furthermore, in clinical studies for evaluating new immunosuppressive drugs or new combinations of drugs, routine graft cytology may help to monitor the efficacy of the therapy and to analyze its immunobiologic effects (Schlitt et al 1992b) which can be helpful for optimal adaptation of a new protocol.

In conclusion, without much harm to the patient a large amount of information about intragraft events can be gathered by routine TAC (Table 4). This information is not only of value for management of the individual patient, but may also help to understand better the physiological and immunological processes that occur in a liver graft following transplantation.

Table 4. Advantages and possibilities of routine monitoring of liver grafts by aspiration cytology

Better interpretation of findings by evaluation of the changes over time

Avoidance of some core biopsies and of "emergency" biopsies

Individual adjustment of immunsuppression in critically ill patients (e.g. during infections)

Evaluation of new immunosuppressive regimens

Material for additional scientific analyses

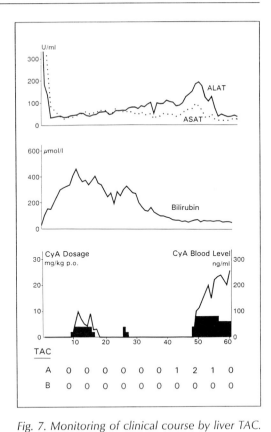

Fig. 7. Monitoring of clinical course by liver TAC. Immunosuppression in this patient had been withdrawn because of severe septic complications and recurrent pneumonia and frequent routine monitoring of the graft was performed by liver TAC. Recurrence of immune activation in the graft by the end of the infectious course was associated with an increase in transaminases indicating the beginning of clinical acute rejection. Reintroduction of basic immunosuppression (cyclosporin and low dose steroids) was sufficient to reverse the rejection process as indicated by rapidly normalizing transaminases and by disappearance of immune activation in the graft.

IMMUNOLOGIC ANALYSES OF INTRAGRAFT EVENTS BY ASPIRATION CYTOLOGY

Apart from the clinically relevant information that is obtained by liver TAC, graft aspirates also yield additional material which can be used for scientific analyses by different methods. For example, cell subpopulations, cell surface markers and other cell associated proteins (cytokines etc.) can be examined by immunocytology using a variety of different antibodies for single or double staining of the cytospin preparations. Similar analyses can be done by flow cytometry using the aspirate as cell suspension, but the number of mononuclear cells is usually too small for adequate flow cytometric evaluation. For detection of specific DNA or RNA in individual cells in situ hybridization is a useful technique, e.g., for detection of graft infection by CMV or other viruses (Arndt et al 1988). Both immunocytology and in situ hybridization can also be applied to cytospin preparations that have been cryopreserved so that retrospective examination of selected patient courses is feasible. Moreover, polymerase chain reaction (PCR) can be used for detection of very small amounts of specific DNA or RNA (own unpublished experience). Quantitation of the findings with this highly sensitive method is still a problem, but semi-quantitative results can be obtained by certain techniques (Dallman et al 1991). Finally, cultivation of the aspirated cells is possible, although the cell numbers are usually too small for direct functional assays. Primary expansion of the cells before functional analysis is, of course, possible, but this probably leads to selection of certain cell populations so that the findings obtained under these conditions may not reflect the actual in vivo situation. Nevertheless, these methods reflect an extensive armamentarium with which the infiltrating cells can be characterized.

The questions addressed by these meth-ods mainly focus on the differentiation of lymphocyte subpopulations present in the graft, their expression of activation markers and adhesion molecules, their T cell receptor repertoire, and their patterns of lymphokine production, and on the surface marker expression of parenchymal cells. In acute rejection, analysis of surface marker expression has shown increased HLA class II and IL-2 receptor (CD25) expression (Lautenschlager et al 1989, Lautenschlager et al 1990) as well as expression of the transferrin receptor (CD71) (Vogel et al 1985). Moreover, an increase in both CD4[+] and CD8[+] T cells was described with the ratio between both cell populations varying over the course of rejection with a predominance of CD4[+] cells early and of CD8[+] cells a few days later (Lautenschlager et al

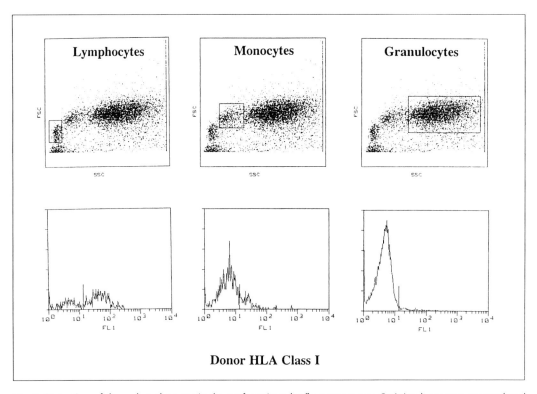

Fig. 8. Detection of donor lymphocytes in the graft aspirate by flow cytometry. Staining by mouse monoclonal antibodies against donor HLA class I (HLA A2) and fluorescein-isothiocyanat-coupled goat-anti-mouse antibody with selective analysis of lymphocytes, monocytes and granulocytes. Gating on different cell populations according to light scatter characteristics (upper row); fluorescence intensity (x-axis) and cell number (y-axis) of these cells (lower row) demonstrating that about two-thirds of the lymphocytes are donor-derived cells, whereas only few monocytes and none of the granulocytes express donor-type HLA class I molecules.

1988a). An increased expression of HLA class I and de novo expression of class II molecules on hepatocytes during rejection has also been observed, but this finding was not specific for rejection (Zannier et al 1988a, Zannier et al 1988b, Steinhoff et al 1988, Vogel et al 1988). In addition, expression of the adhesion molecule ICAM-1 on hepatocytes has been shown to appear early in the course of clinical rejection, even before clinical manifestation (Lautenschlager et al 1992), but due the low specificity of this finding it is also not very helpful for preclinical diagnosis and early treatment of rejection. There is also some evidence that the extent and pattern of activation marker expression on mononuclear cells and on hepatocytes is influenced considerably by the immunosuppressive regimen applied.

Since the interactions between the populations of infiltrating lymphocytes with each other and with the different parenchymal cells represent a highly complex network, the serial analysis of the receptor repertoire of the involved T lymphocytes, their cytokine production profile, and the expression of molecules involved in cell-cell interactions in sequential graft aspirates may help to uncover the immunological processes occurring in the graft. The findings obtained from such analysis can, thus, help to understand the in vivo function and the pharmacodynamics of the various drugs and drug combinations so that immunosuppressive regimens may be optimized not only by evaluating their clinical effects but on a better defined immunological basis.

Another finding that was made by routine aspiration cytology is that lymphocytes of the liver donor can obviously persist in the graft for about two weeks after transplantation (Fig. 8). There is some evidence that these donor lymphocytes may be involved in immune processes in the graft that resemble rejection-like immune activation morphologically but that are not associated with clinical rejection (Schlitt et al 1993b). Whether the immune activation observed in these situations is caused by a localized slight graft-versus-host activity or whether it represents an alloresponse of the recipient that is somehow modulated by the donor lymphocytes remains to be clarified. The persistence of donor lymphocytes in the graft early after transplantation, however, adds another facet to the already complex immune network in the graft.

CURRENT STATE AND PERSPECTIVES OF LIVER TAC

Growing experience with the method has shown that transplant aspiration cytology can be very helpful for clinical management of liver-grafted patients, particularly if it is used as monitoring method. Its main strength lies in its ability to follow intragraft immune events and it could be shown that a typical immune activation in the graft is necessary but not sufficient for the diagnosis of acute graft rejection. The method has several advantages but it also has clear limits which must be respected in order to avoid overinterpretation. It also must be kept in mind that the information obtained by aspiration cytology represents only one small aspect of the overall morphology and pathophysiology of the graft. Although the biopsy material can be—and has been—analyzed by a variety of immunological methods, so far routine hematologic staining is sufficient for clinical practice.

The future aims with the method are a more precise characterization of the immunologic state of the graft than can be obtained by mere gross description of immune activation, e.g., by an analysis of cytokine profiles in the graft and by receptor analysis of the infiltrating lymphocytes. Such studies would help to delineate the complex network-like functional interactions between the different cell types that occur after allogeneic organ transplantation. Besides a better evaluation and optimization of immunosuppressive treatment such analyses might probably also help in the definition of tolerance-like states for the graft which would facilitate individual adaptation, i.e., particularly reduction, in immunosuppression in individual graft recipients.

REFERENCES

Arndt R, Heinzer H, Hammerer P, Huland H, Löhning T, Krämer-Hansen H (1988). Identification of virus DNA in kidney tranplants by fine-needle aspiration biopsy. Transplant Proc 1988 20:581.

Carbonnel F, Samuel D, Reynes M, Benhamou JP, Bismuth H, Bach JF, Chatenoud L (1990). Fine-needle aspiration biopsy of human liver allografts. Correlation with liver histology for the diagnosis of acute rejection. Transplantation 50:704.

Dallman MJ, Larsen CP, Morris PJ (1991). Cytokine gene transcription in vascularized organ grafts: analysis using semiquantitative polymerase chain reaction. J Exp Med 174:493.

Fehrman I, Greene C, Tillery W (1988). Transplant aspiration cytology for diagnosis of liver allograft rejection. Transplant Proc 20:657.

Greene CL, Fehrman I, Tillery GW, Husberg BS, Klintmalm GB (1988a). A clear distinction between "immune activation of rejection" and "no immune activation" in liver transplant aspiration cytology. Transplant Proc 20:661.

Greene CL, Parker DM, Bramley AR (1988b). A rapid Romanowsky stain for transplant cytology specimens. Transplant Proc 20:573.

Greene CL, Fehrman I, Tillery GW, Husberg BS, Klintmalm GB (1988c). Liver transplant aspiration cytology is useful for monitoring steroid treatment of rejection. Transplant Proc 20:659.

Häyry P, von Willebrand E (1981). Practical guidelines for fine needle aspiration biopsy of human renal allografts. Ann Clin Res 13:288.

Kirby RM, Young JA, Hübscher SG, Elias S, McMaster P (1988). The accuracy of aspiration cytology in the diagnosis of rejection following orthotopic liver transplantation. Transplant Int 1:119.

Kubota K, Ericzon BG, Reinholt FP (1991). Comparison of fine-needle aspiration biopsy and histology in human liver transplants. Transplantation 51:1010.

Lautenschlager I, Höckerstedt K, Ahonen J, Eklund B, Isoniemi H, Korsbäck C, Pettersson E, Salmela K, Scheinin TM, von Willebrand E, Häyry P (1988a). Fine-needle aspiration biopsy in the monitoring of liver allografts. II.

Application to human liver allografts. Transplantation 46:47.

Lautenschlager I, Höckerstedt K, Taskinen E, Korsbäck C, Mäkisalo H, Häyry P (1988b). Fine-needle aspiration biopsy in the monitoring of liver allografts. I. Correlation between aspiration biopsy and core biopsy in experimental pig liver allografts. Transplantation 46:41.

Lautenschlager I, Höckerstedt K, Häyry P (1989). Correlation of cytological findings to activation markers in acute liver rejection. Transplant Proc 21:2290.

Lautenschlager I, Höckerstedt K, Salmela K, Isoniemi H, Holmberg C, Jalanko H, Häyry P (1990). Fine-needle aspiration biopsy in the monitoring of liver allografts. Different cellular findings during rejection and cytomegalovirus infection. Transplantation 50:798.

Lautenschlager I, Höckerstedt K, Häyry P (1991). Fine-needle aspiration biopsy in the monitoring of liver allografts. Transplant Int 4:54.

Lautenschlager I, Höckerstedt K, Häyry P (1992). Intercellular adhesion molecule 1 (ICAM-1) induction on hepatocytes is an early marker for acute liver allograft rejection. Transplant Int 5(Suppl.1):S283.

Ludwig J (1988). Histopathology of the liver following transplantation. In: Maddrey WC, ed. Current topics in gastroenterology: Transplantation of the liver. New York: Elsevier p.191.

Nashan B, Schlitt HJ, Wittekind C, Ringe B, Wonigeit K, Pichlmayr R (1989). Patterns of immune activation during the first four weeks in liver transplanted patients. Transplant Proc 21:3623.

Nashan B, Schlitt HJ, Ringe B, Bunzendahl H, Wonigeit K, Pichlmayr R (1990). Transplantation aspiration cytology in the diagnosis of steroid resistant rejection in liver allografted patients. Transplant Proc 22:2297.

Nashan B, Schlitt HJ, Ringe B, Bunzendahl H, Wittekind C, Wonigeit K, Pichlmayr R (1991). Differential diagnosis of viral infections and acute rejection episodes in liver grafted patients by transplant aspiration cytology. Transplant Proc 23:1507.

Pasternack A, Virolainen M, Häyry P (1973). Fine needle aspiration biopsy in the diagnosis of human renal allograft rejection. J Urol 109:167.

Portmann B, Wight DGD (1987). Pathology of liver transplantation (excluding rejection). In: Calne RY, ed. Liver transplantation: the Cambridge/King's College Hospital experience. London: Grune & Stratton, p.437.

Schlitt HJ, Nashan B, Ringe B, Wittekind C, Wonigeit K, Pichlmayr R (1989). Clinical usefulness of a semiquantitative scoring sysstem for liver transplant aspiration cytology. Transplant Proc 21:3621.

Schlitt HJ, Nashan B, Ringe B, Bunzendahl H, Wittekind C, Wonigeit K, Pichlmayr R (1991a). Differentiation of liver graft dysfunction by transplant aspiration cytology. Transplantation 51:786.

Schlitt HJ, Nashan B, Krick P, Ringe B, Bunzendahl H, Wittekind C, Wonigeit K, Pichlmayr R (1991b). Acute liver graft rejection: correlation between morphological and clinical diagnosis. In: Engemann R, Hamelmann H, eds. Experimental and clinical liver transplantation. Amsterdam: Elsevier Science, p.31.

Schlitt HJ, Nashan B, Krick P, Ringe B, Wittekind C, Wonigeit K, Pichlmayr R (1992a). Intragraft immune events after human liver transplantation. Correlation with clinical signs of acute rejection and influence of immunosuppression. Transplantation 54:273.

Schlitt HJ, Nashan B, Ringe B, Wonigeit K, Pichlmayr R (1992b). Subclinical acute rejection after liver transplantation: incidence, clinical relevance and effect of immunosuppression. In: Shapira Z, Yussim A, Hammer C, eds. Transplant monitoring. Lengerich: Wolfgang Pabst Verlag, 225.

Schlitt HJ, Nashan B, Ringe B, Wonigeit K, Pichlmayr R (1993a). Routine monitoring of liver grafts by transplant aspiration cytology (TAC)—clinical experience with 3,000 TACs. Transplant Proc 251:1970.

Schlitt HJ, Kanehiro H, Raddatz G, Steinhoff G, Richter N, Nashan B, Ringe B, Wonigeit K, Pichlmayr R. (1993b). Persistence of donor

lymphocytes in liver allograft recipients. Transplantation (in press).

Snover DC, Freese DK, Sharp HL, Bloomer JR, Najarian JS, Ascher NL (1987). Liver allograft rejection. An analysis of the use of biopsy determining outcome of rejection. Am J Surg Pathol 11:1.

Steinhoff G, Wonigeit K, Pichlmayr R (1988). Analysis of sequential changes in major histocompatibility complex expression in human liver grafts after transplantation. Transplantation 45:394.

Vogel W, Margreiter R, Schmalzl F, Judmaier G (1984). Preliminary results with fine needle aspiration biopsy in liver grafts. Transplant Proc 16:1240.

Vogel W, Portman B, Williams R (1985). Difference of OKT9 antigen expression in rejection aspiration biopsies from human liver grafts. Transplant Proc 20:648.

Vogel W, Wohlfahrter P, Then P, Judmaier G, Knapp W, Margreiter R (1988). Longitudinal study of major histocompatibility complex antigen expression on hepatocytes in fine-needle aspiration biopsies from human liver grafts. Transplant Proc 20:648.

Wight DGD, Portmann B (1987). Pathology of liver transplantation. In: Calne RY, ed. Liver transplantation: the Cambridge/King's College Hospital experience. London: Grune & Stratton, p.385.

von Willebrand E, Häyry P (1984). Reproducibility of fine needle aspiration biopsy. Analysis of 93 double biopsies. Transplantation 38:314.

Zannier A, Faure JL, Mutin M, Champetier P, Takvorian P, Neidecker J (1988a). Aspiration cytology of liver allografts: monitoring of hepatocyte major histocompatibility complex-DR expression increases accuracy of diagnosis of rejection episodes. Transplantation Proc 20:650.

Zannier A, Pujol B, Berger F, Paliard P (1988b). Characterization of cellular infiltrate and HLA-DR expression in chronic hepatitis B-virus infection using fine-needle aspiration cytology. Transplant Proc 20:652.

================CHAPTER 3================

ACCELERATED REJECTION OF LIVER GRAFTS WITH PARTICULAR ATTENTION TO FK506

Ignazio Roberto Marino, Thomas E. Starzl, John J. Fung

INTRODUCTION

Vascularized organ transplants can be rejected by either humoral or cell mediated mechanisms that are not mutually exclusive. This is not unexpected given the relation of both arms of the immune system. Cell mediated rejection in naive recipients of allografts is a first set immune event, generally requiring days to development of cellular rejection. Yet, donor specific antibodies can be detected in allografts which are undergoing first set rejection. On the other hand, proliferative and cytotoxic donor specific T cell responses can be detected in vitro in animals which have been presensitized to donor antigens. Isolated reports of accelerated cell mediated rejection exist in sensitized recipients, (Eichwald et al 1985) but overall this is uncommon, and the focus of this chapter will be to discuss the role of antibodies in accelerated liver transplant rejection.

CHARACTERIZATION OF ANTIBODIES INVOLVED IN REJECTION

The phenomenon of hyperacute rejection was first recognized as being related to preformed antibodies in kidney allografts transplanted in ABO incompatible combinations. These findings were also noted in recipients bearing lymphocytotoxic antibodies, as a result of pregnancy, previous blood transfusions or failed grafts. The importance of avoiding transplantation of kidney allografts into recipients bearing preformed antidonor antibodies was noted in many early reports describing hyperacute rejection (Starzl 1964, Terasaki et al 1965, Kissmeyer-Nielsen et al 1966, Williams et al 1968, Starzl et al 1970). The impact of preformed antibodies in other vascularized organ allografts is variable, with the heart being susceptible to antibody rejection, (Rose 1991) while the liver is less vulnerable. (Starzl 1969, 1974, 1987, Garnier 1965, 1970, Cordier 1966, Calne 1967a, b, 1969, 1970a, Peacock 1967, Lempinen 1971, Mazzoni 1971, Iwatsuki 1981, 1984, Houssin 1985,

1986, Orosz 1986, Gordon 1986a, Gubernatis 1987, Knechtle 1987a, b, Gugenheim 1988a, b, Demetris 1988, 1989, Davies 1989, Suminoto 1991, Furuya in press).

In xenotransplantation, preformed antibodies occur naturally, without prior exposure to antigens from other species of animals. These antibodies are capable of mediating a brisk hyperacute rejection (Perper 1966a, b, Calne 1970b, Giles 1970). It is thought that these naturally occurring antibodies are the results of exposure to common environmental antigens (Marino 1990, First 1992). These antibodies react with glycolipids and glycoproteins on the cell surface of the xenograft.

The class of immunoglobulins involved in hyperacute rejection depends on the antigenic determinants which the antibodies recognize. Lymphocytotoxic antibodies to MHC determinants, as a result of prior transfusion or failed allografts, are often of the IgG class. Both xenoantibodies and, to a great extent, ABO isoagglutinins are of the IgM class, but high titers of IgG can be induced by sensitization. The titer of preformed xenoantibodies and ease of inducing xenoantibodies was proposed to be able to provide an assessment of phylogenic diversity (Landsteiner 1962), hence the designation of discordant and concordant combinations (Calne 1970b).

In the discordant xenotransplant combination, IgM and IgG can be shown to exist in high titers, such as in the guinea pig-to-rat combination (Gambiez 1990), the pig-to-Rhesus monkey combination (Fischel 1990) and the pig-to-dog combination (Giles 1970, Makowka 1987). In concordant xenotransplant combinations IgM may exist, usually in low titers, such as in the hamster-to-rat combination (Valdivia 1987a), the fox-to-dog combination (Brendel 1977), and baboon-to-rhesus monkey combination (Marquet 1978). In both combinations, sensitization following transplantation generally results in an abrupt rise in the IgM titer followed shortly by an increase in the IgG titer. In a few models, other classes of immunoglobulins besides IgG and IgM, can cause hyperacute rejection. In some of our previous experimental studies, IgA and IgG were able to initiate hyperacute rejection in a kidney transplant model (Marino 1990, 1991).

PATHOPHYSIOLOGY OF ANTIBODY MEDIATED REJECTION

Independent of the nature of immunoglobulin class of preformed antibody involved in triggering antibody mediated rejection, the pathophysiology of the acute inflammatory response is similar. Preformed antibodies trigger rejection by their deposition on the endothelium of the vascularized graft. These antibodies in turn activate complement, which in turn activates a characteristic cascade of inflammatory, nonspecific mediators, such as recruitment of polymorphonuclear leukocytes, platelet adhesion and degranulation, followed by intravascular thrombosis (Starzl 1964, Kissmeyer-Nielsen 1966, Williams 1968, Giles 1970) (Figs. 1 and 2).

Complement activation can occur via the classical and alternative complement pathways. In the classical pathway, the C1q component of C1 is activated following binding to the Fc region of IgM and IgG. This in turn results in C1r and C1s activation and the generation of the C1qrs protease complex, in turn leading to C4 and C2 cleavage, producing the C3 convertase, C4b2a complex. C3 is then cleaved to produce the biologically active components, C3a and C3b. In the alternative pathway, complement can be activated via IgA, IgE and other nonimmunologic factors such as polysaccharides and bacteria. Activation of C3 occurs via nonspecific cleavage to generate C3b.

The common pathway of complement activation is via the C5 cleavage which generates C5b which in turn leads to the assembly of the C5b-C9 membrane attack complex. This membrane attack complex binds to the cell surface resulting in a porous membrane which is susceptible to osmotic pressure leading to either cell damage or cell death.

Cell damage also occurs by activation of other inflammatory pathways. Reactive oxygen metabolites, prostaglandins and cytokines can be generated by the degradation products of complement activation (Forbes 1982). Polymorphonuclear leukocytes and macrophages are attracted to the site of inflammation via the C5a fragment, which results in the release of lysosomal enzymes and resultant cell damage (Forbes 1984). C3b also enhances adhesion of these cells to damage cells. C3b also promotes binding of platelets which may lead to degranulation and release of vasoactive substances, such as serotonin and histamine, both increasing vascular permeability.

Thrombosis of the microvasculature is enhanced by the loss of membrane associated heparin sulfate, from the endothelial cell. The release of tissue factors from injured cells also promotes thrombosis.

The importance of complement in the pathophysiology of antibody mediated rejection is shown in studies in which complement is depleted. Cobra venom inactivates the C3 component, resulting in paralysis of the complement system (Kemp 1982, Adachi 1987, Johnston 1992). Hasan and coworkers have been able to obtain long-term survival of xenografts during treatment with cobra venom factor (Hasan 1992).

SUSCEPTIBILITY OF THE LIVER TO ANTIBODY MEDICATED REJECTION

Transplanted livers have been reported to be relatively resistant to both cell mediated and antibody mediated rejection (Starzl 1969, 1974, 1987, Garnier 1965, 1970, Cordier 1966, Calne 1967a, b, 1969, 1970a, Peacock 1967, Lempinen 1971, Mazzoni 1971, Iwatsuki 1981, 1984, Houssin 1985, 1986, Gordon 1986a, Orosz 1986, Gubernatis 1987, Knechtle 1987a,b, Gugenheim 1988a,b, Demetris 1988, 1989, Davies 1989, Suminoto 1991, Furuya, in press). Liver allografts were shown to have prolonged survival when compared to organs and tissues, when immuno-

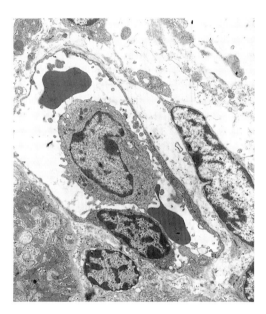

Fig. 1. Electron photomicrograph of a xenografted kidney (pig-to-rabbit) tissue sample obtained 15 minutes after reperfusion. In the peritubular capillary a monocyte, erythrocytes and platelets (showing some adherence to the endothelium) can be observed. The interstitium is edematous (x4600). (Reprinted from : Histopathological, immunofluorescent, and electron-microscopic features of hyperacute rejection in discordant renal xenotransplantation, by Marino IR et al, in Xenotransplantation, Cooper DKC, Kemp E, Reemtsma K, and White DJG eds., Springer-Verlag, Berlin, Chapter 12, Fig. 12.6, p.214, 1991).

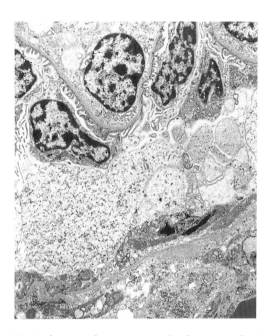

Fig. 2. Electron photomicrograph of a xenografted kidney (pig-to-rabbit) tissue sample obtained 120 minutes after reperfusion. The urinary space of the glomerulus is completely occupied by cell debris, and the epithelial cells of the Bowman's capsule are dramatically damaged (x4600). (Reprinted from: Histopathological, immunofluorescent, and electron-microscopic features of hyperacute rejection in discordant renal xenotransplantation, by Marino IR et al, in Xenotransplantation, Cooper DKC, Kemp E, Reemtsma K, and White DJG eds., Springer-Verlag, Berlin, Chapter 12, Fig. 12.15, p.223, 1991).

suppression is not given. In fact, several groups have demonstrated spontaneous liver allograft survival in the porcine model, without immunosuppression (Calne 1967a, b, Peacock 1967, Lempinen 1971, Mazzoni 1971).

A number of observations on the effect of the presensitized state on liver transplant survival suggests that the liver is less susceptible to antibody mediated rejection. Starzl and coworkers have noted resistance of human liver allografts to humoral rejection (Starzl 1974, Iwatsuki 1981, 1984). This resistance is sufficient to allow transplantation under conditions which would be unacceptable for kidneys. It has been evident that hyperacute rejection of the liver does not commonly occur with lymphocytotoxic presensitized states, while occurring more frequently with ABO-incompatible liver transplants. While a penalty accrues to those patients receiving ABO-incompatible liver allografts, there were a surprisingly large number of such grafts that were successful (Starzl 1974, 1987, Iwatsuki 1981, 1984, Gordon 1986a, Demetris 1988, 1989, 1992, Rego 1987, Gugenheim 1989, 1990, Fischel 1989). The pathology of the ABO-mismatched livers which failed revealed evidence of humoral rejection, with hemorrhagic necrosis and intraparenchymal coagulation (Demetris 1988, 1989). The long-term complication of ABO-incompatibility may also manifest with biliary tract complications (Starzl 1987, Demetris 1989, Sanchez-Urdazpal 1991). This pattern of rejection is rarely seen in liver allografts in which a positive lymphocytotoxic crossmatch occurs. As would be predicted, the pattern of xenoantibody rejection of the liver is much more similar to that of ABO-incompatibility than for MHC specific sensitization. In animals receiving a discordant liver transplant, IgM and IgG deposition on the vascular endothelium and sinusoids is also accompanied by complement activation. Vascular thrombosis due to platelet aggregation leads to hemorrhagic necrosis, with little or no cellular infiltrates.

The relative resistance of the liver allograft to antibody mediated rejection appears to confer some protection systemically, presumably by neutralizing or reducing the titer of lymphocytotoxic antibodies. One of the possible explanations for this unique capacity of the liver to withstand antibody attack is the observation that the liver is a source of soluble MHC Class I antigens (Davies 1989, Suminoto 1991). These soluble MHC antigens may neutralize the circulating antidonor antibody (Houssin 1985, 1986, Orosz 1986, Gugenheim 1988a, b). In addition, the liver serves as a rich reticuloendothelial organ, removing circulating immune complexes by actions of the Kupffer cell which lines a nonendothelial vascular network which is less susceptible to vasoactive substances than endorgan vessels such as seen with the heart and kidney.

Extracorporeal donor-specific liver hemoperfusion can reduce the level of cytotoxic antibodies in hypersensitized rats (Orosz 1986, Gugenheim 1985, 1988, Kamada 1988). This finding was the premise to utilize the liver allograft to protect the subsequent kidney allograft in patients with preformed donor-specific antibodies (Fung 1988, Flye 1990). The lymphocytotoxic crossmatch in patients with preformed antibodies will often convert from positive to negative following liver transplantation. When this occurs, placement of a kidney allograft from the same donor will often result in prevention of hyperacute rejection of the kidney (Fung 1988, Flye 1990). It should be noted that this protection is not universal, and cases of rejection of the kidney following liver transplantation have been reported (Starzl 1989).

In spite of the unique immunologic properties of the liver, reports of accelerated rejection of the liver have been published (Hanto 1987, Bird 1989, Starzl 1989, Karuppan 1991). Knechtle and coworkers noted that the resistance of liver allografts to rejection could be overridden by presensitization with skin grafts (Knechtle 1987a,b). In 9 of 10 presensitized rat recipients, hyperacute rejection was noted, and immunofluorescence could detect IgG and complement in the sinusoids and perivascular tissues. Murase and coworkers also noted antibody mediated rejection in an arterialized rat liver transplant model if the recipients had received at least four skin grafts from the donor, and if the transplant was performed within nine weeks (Furuya in press). In a porcine model of acceptance of liver allografts, the liver allograft could be induced to be uniformly rejected when the recipient pigs were presensitized, either by prior skin grafting or kidney transplantation (Calne 1969). In a primate study, Gubernatis and coworkers demonstrated that hyperacute or accelerated rejection of the liver could be observed (Gubernatis 1987).

The first report of hemorrhagic necrosis following human liver transplantation was by Williams and Hume, more than 25 years ago (Hume 1969). In 1987, Hanto and coworkers published a case report of hyperacute rejection in a strongly positive T cell crossmatched recipient (Hanto 1987). The pattern of rejection in this patient was notable for a lack of antibody and complement in the sinusoids or portal vessels. The adverse effect of lymphocytotoxic antibodies in liver allograft survival in human liver transplantation may have been masked by the immunosuppression which has been utilized in most immunosuppressive regimens. In contrast to the early reports on the relative lack of effect of a positive crossmatch on liver allograft survival (Iwatsuki 1981, 1984), Takaya and coworkers noted that there was an increased graft loss in these patients (Takaya 1992a). The principle difference in the two populations was the utilization of high dose steroids in the former group, while low dose steroids (20 mg/day) were utilized in the latter group. In fact, when the steroid doses were increased in subsequent positive crossmatch liver recipients, the incidence of graft loss decreased.

TREATMENT OF THE PREFORMED ANTIBODY STATE

Since 1956 a number of treatments have been proposed as methods to reduce preformed antibodies, or to minimize the damage which would be antibody mediated (Clark 1964, 1966, Gerwurz 1966, Rosenberg 1969, 1971a, b, Shons 1970, 1973, 1974a, b, Bier 1970, Moberg 1971, Hawkins 1971, Kux 1971, Merkel 1971, Baldamus 1973, Winn 1973, Kemp 1982, 1976, 1977, 1987a, b, Shapiro 1990a). These include:

antibody depletion (including specific and nonspecific antibody removal), interruption of the clotting cascade, and interruption of the complement cascade.

Several antibody depletion techniques have been utilized in the past 30 years. The first report of thoracic duct drainage (TDD) was in 1964 (Franksson 1964, 1967, 1976). A number of series of patients treated with TDD in the pre-cyclosporine era, undergoing kidney transplantation, have been reported (Sonoda 1966, Murray 1968, Tilney 1968, 1970, Archimbaud 1969, Martelli 1970, Sarles 1970, Estevam 1974, Walker 1977, Johnson 1977, Starzl 1979a, b, Koep 1980, Ono 1987, Ohshima 1981, 1987, 1988, 1989c, d). In these series, it was noted that the level of lymphocytotoxic antibodies fell during the course of TDD. However, with the advent of cyclosporine, the cumbersome use of TDD has been largely abandoned.

Plasmapheresis has also been utilized to lower preformed antibody levels. This technique has also been combined with cyclophosphamide, an antiproliferative agent (Marino 1993), in highly sensitized patients receiving kidney transplants (Taube 1984a, b). Its use in the posttransplant period to reverse established antibody rejection has met with varying success (Cardella 1977, Naik 1979, Rifle 1979, Kirubakaran 1981, Power 1981). The cost and variable efficacy has also led to abandonment of this procedure.

A relatively newly described method to lower antibody levels is the ability of the *Staphylococcus aureus* Protein A to bind to the Fc receptor of IgG (Forsgren 1966). The application of this principle to column technology has allowed Protein A to be bound covalently to cyanogen bromide activated Sepharose B, creating a solid phase immunoabsorbant. It has been possible to deplete serum IgG levels by 75-90% with a single treatment (Shapiro 1990a). Few clinical trials have been performed both in Europe and in the United States, and the results have also been variable (Palmer 1987, 1989, Gjorstrup 1988, Shapiro 1990b.)

The use of antigen-specific antibody depletion has centered on the pre-perfusion of a donor vascularized organ prior to transplantation. Reports by Starzl and coworkers with pre-perfusion of liver, kidneys and spleen by heterotopic ex vivo perfusion of the recipient, was shown to immediately decrease the levels of preformed antibodies (Giles 1970). This allowed prolonged graft survival in situations which normally would lead to rejection.

Other techniques to control the damage mediated by preformed antibodies have focused on abrogating the inflammatory mediator response (Makowka 1987), interrupting the clotting cascade (Giles 1970, 1971, Kux 1971, Moberg 1971, Kemp 1976, 1977, 1982), or preventing complement activation (Moberg 1971, Kemp 1982, Adachi 1987, Johnston 1992, Hasan 1992). Unfortunately, none of these techniques have resulted in clinical applications. Inhibition of soluble mediators with antiplatelet activating factors have provided encouraging laboratory results, especially if combined with prostaglandins, but generally at the expense of an hemorrhagic diathesis. Kux and coworkers described the use of a calcium chelating agent, sodium citrate, over 20 years ago (Kux 1971). Citrate theoretically functions by virtue of its anticoagulation ability, but also secondarily by inhibition of complement activation, which is also calcium dependent. In this model, citrate was perfused intra-arterially into the vascularized organ. Unfortunately, the doses of citrate which are required, soon led to citrate intoxication.

Prevention of complement activation is a strategy which is attractive for future development. Cobra venom, which was described over 20 years ago for its ability to prevent complement activation, is also a potent anticoagulant. It has been effective in prolonging the hyperacute rejection of guinea pig hearts in a discordant xenograft model using rats as recipients (Johnston 1992).

USE OF FK506 IN PRESENSITIZED STATES

Nonspecific immunosuppression has been utilized to decrease the immune responsiveness in preformed antibody states. Many of these agents have required "cocktail" therapy, including agents which act on different limbs of the immune response (Murase 1993, in

press). Cyclosporine has not been very effective in the xenograft models (Adachi 1987, Valdivia 1987b, Gambiez 1990). On the other hand, another T cell specific immunosuppressive agent, FK506, has some effect in xenograft models, in which the level of preformed antibodies is low (Valdivia 1987a).

FK506 is a newly described macrolide antibiotic, with potent suppression of both cell mediated and T cell dependent antibody responses (Kino 1987, Starzl 1991).

The large experience accumulated in the last four years with the clinical use of FK506 showed very encouraging results (Starzl 1991) when compared with the other drugs presently used. However, limited information is available on the effect of FK506 on the humoral response, both experimentally and clinically. In 1988, Woo et al (Woo 1988), demonstrated profound suppression of the production of splenic IgM-secreting plasma cells and antibody levels in rats immunized with sheep red blood cells. IgM-producing splenic plasma cells underwent a 93% reduction in the group of animals treated with FK506 in association with cyclosporine, and a 98% reduction in the group treated with FK506 alone. Inamura et al (Inamura 1988), that same year, and Takagishi et al (Takagishi 1989), the following year, showed that when FK506 treatment was begun on the same day as type II collagen immunization, FK506 inhibited the development of arthritis and suppressed and immunological response to type II collagen in rats. These findings, along with the fact that experimental arthritis can be induced in congenitally athymic nude rats by humoral mechanism alone (Takagishi 1985), can be explained as a result of the inhibition of anticollagen antibody production by FK506.

Our group has reported in the past (Iwatsuki 1981, 1984, Gordon 1986b) that one and two year liver graft survivals were not adversely affected by the lymphocytotoxic antibody and that a positive crossmatch was not a contraindication for liver transplantation. However, the fact that many of the crossmatch positive patients were highly sensitized and that specific alloimmunization of platelets to class I antigens is a major cause of bleeding and platelet transfusion refractoriness in liver transplant candidates was documented shortly thereafter (Marino 1988). These facts, along with the knowledge that crossmatch-positive liver grafts have been lost for unclear reasons (Hanto 1987, Bird 1989, Starzl 1989, Karuppan 1991) in different centers motivated us to reanalyze the effect of antidonor lymphocytotoxic antibody upon graft survival. Takaya et al demonstrated, for the first time and in the largest patient series available, that antidonor lymphocytotoxic antibody (positive crossmatch) adversely affects the survival of primary liver transplantation during the first 12 months after surgery (Fig. 3) (Takaya 1991, 1992a). These studies showed an increased incidence of graft failure from rejection, and of vascular and biliary complications in this population. The adverse impact of using positive cytotoxic crossmatch donors was evident both under cyclosporine or FK506 as primary immunosuppressant (Takaya 1991, 1992a). There was no difference in the one-year graft survival between 25 positive crossmatch patients in the FK506 era (56%), when compared to 22 positive crossmatch patients in the cyclosporine era (59%) (Takaya 1991, 1992a). Similar results in a series of liver transplant patients have been also reported by Karuppan et al in Sweden (Karuppan 1991). None of the grafts in this Swedish series were hyperacutely rejected, and graft survival was significantly lower in the group of patients that had cytotoxic antibodies reactive with donor splenic T and/or B cells. Nakamura et al (Nakamura 1991) conducted a clinicopathologic analysis of 26 liver transplant recipients harboring preformed dithiothreitol (DTT) resistant (Iwaki 1988) lymphocytotoxic antibodies. These 26 patients were identified among adult patients who received primary liver allografts under FK506 immunosuppression at the University of Pittsburgh. Similar to the smaller Swedish series, none of the grafts of this Pittsburgh series underwent "hyperacute" rejection. On the

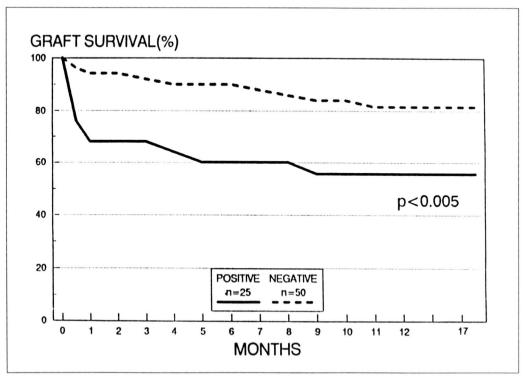

Fig. 3. The actuarial graft survival rates in 25 adult liver transplant positive-crossmatch patients and 50 negative-crossmatch patients (Reprinted from: The adverse impact on liver transplantation of using positive cytotoxic crossmatch donors, by Takaya S. et al, in Transplantation 53(2):p.401, Fig.1, 1992).

other hand, when compared to crossmatch negative control patients, the crossmatch positive recipients had prolonged early graft dysfunction, a significantly larger number of clinically indicated biopsies, and of biopsy proven early acute cellular rejection within the first 10 post transplant days. There was also a higher incidence of graft failure within the first two months. Furthermore, pathologic specimens from these positive crossmatch patients showed early platelet margination in central veins and sinusoids, neutrophilic portal venulitis followed by cholangiolar proliferation, acute cholangiolitis, centrilobular hepatocyte swelling (mimicking "preservation" injury), relapsing episodes of acute cellular rejection and endothelial activation of arteries with medial changes. A significant clinical difference in the course of these patients is represented by the fact that the centrilobular hepatocyte swelling mimicking a "preservation" injury often do not resolve (as generally happens in the "true" preservation injury) but rather tend to persist or worsen in the posttransplant weeks. All these pathologic events indicated that transplant recipients harboring preformed DTT-resistant lymphocytotoxic antibodies have a worse early posttransplantation graft function and survival, even though in these FK506-treated recipients hyperacute or accelerated rejection was not seen. These clinicopathologic results were actually very similar to the experimental observations by Houssin et al (Houssin 1985, 1986), and Furuya et al (Furuya in press). In fact, the seven (27%) failed allografts from crossmatch positive patients in the Pittsburgh series showed significant changes in the arteries and in the peribiliary vascular plexus (Nakamura 1991). The medium-sized muscular arteries presented changes suggestive of arterial spasm (Nakamura 1991), resembling the changes observed in sensitized rats (Furuya in press). Also, medial thickening was common and an analysis of the arterial wall thickness/diameter ratio resulted in a significant difference between the crossmatch positive patients and the controls. Immunofluorescence revealed venous and sinusoidal IgG, C1q, and C3 deposition only in biopsies performed 6-24 hours after liver reperfusion (Iwaki 1988). No signifi-

cant immune deposits were detectable later in biopsy specimens. This was the only important dissimilarity between the clinical (Nakamura 1991) and the experimental (Furuya in press) pathologic findings.

Differing from renal grafts, where humoral rejection does not respond to immunosuppression, there is clinical evidence that sensitized liver allograft recipients may resist an antibody-mediated rejection if an FK506 based immune suppression regimen is used (Woodle 1991, Takaya 1992b). Woodle et al (Woodle 1991) reported a case of biopsy proven liver humoral rejection, where an ABO-incompatible donor organ was used (A to O), that promptly resolved after switching the patient to FK506 immunosuppression. Initial posttransplant liver biopsies showed several features of humoral rejection, including arteriolar hyaline necrosis, disrupted endothelium, intraluminal fibrin deposition, and IgM and complement endothelial deposition. All these findings regressed four days after FK506 treatment was started and disappeared in eight days. Even though plasmapheresis and OKT3 were used perioperatively the clinicopathologic picture dramatically improved only when FK506 therapy was initiated, unequivocally supporting the use of this drug in a similar condition.

More recently, Takaya et al (Takaya 1992b) reported their experience in positive cytotoxic crossmatch liver transplant patients using FK506 in conjunction with high dose steroids and prostaglandin E_1 (PGE_1) (Quagliata 1972, Mundy 1980, Rappaport 1982, Strom 1983, Shaw 1985, Makowka 1987, Starzl 1993, Marino 1993). Using this immunosuppressive strategy it was possible to convert the prognosis of recipients harboring preformed cytotoxic antibodies to essentially the same as that of the conventionally treated crossmatch negative recipients. In fact, the six-month graft survival rate in the positive crossmatch patients treated with low dose steroids was only 60.7%, while the six-month graft survival rate in the group treated with high dose steroids and PGE_1 was 92.9% (P=0.03). This Pittsburgh study, along with the experience reported by Woodle et al (Woodle 1991) indicates that it is possible under FK506 treatment to transplant a liver into a sensitized recipient with a reasonable expectation of avoiding accelerated or hyperacute rejection. However, long-term results are needed before it can be concluded that the strengthened immuno- suppression can ameliorate the effects of preformed antibodies to the point that this should not be considered an issue. A longer clinicopathologic followup should clarify if the better short-term results are not subsequently diminished by biliary or vascular complications like biliary sludge, bile duct necrosis or small bile duct loss. These could appear later and nevertheless be the result of an initial antibody mediated damage. If the long-term follow-up does not show an increased incidence of any of these complications a positive crossmatch or an ABO-incompatibility would not be considered an absolute contraindication to liver transplantation in the FK506 era. Especially considering the observation of "mutual natural immunosuppression" that is established between the donor and the recipient by the donor-recipient cell traffic starting immediately after reperfusion (Iwaki 1991). Recently, Starzl and Demetris (Starzl submitted) stated, on the basis of the Pittsburgh investigations on mixed allogeneic microchimerism that "if the initial storm can be weathered, as has been increasingly possible with modern immunosuppression, the anticipated typing effect dwindles". Most probably FK506, along with "old" immunosuppressive drugs (steroids, PGE_1, cyclophosphamide) (Marino 1993, Starzl 1993) and possible manipulation of immune cells effecting the microchimeric state (Monaco 1970, Caridis 1973, Slavin 1977, Thomas 1983, Ildstad 1985, Barber 1991, Starzl submitted) will allow the antibody barrier in allo- and xenotransplantations to be routinely overcome.

Acknowledgements

We would like to express our gratitude to Howard R. Doyle, M.D. and Cataldo Doria, M.D., for reviewing the chapter and for their advice. We also wish to thank Linda Buckley for her valuable assistance in preparing the manuscript.

References

Adachi H, Rosengard BR, Hutchins GM, Hall TS, Baumgartner WA, Borkon AM, Reitz BA (1987). Effects of cyclosporine, aspirin, and cobra venom factor on discordant cardiac xenograft survival in rats. Transplant Proc, 19:1145-1148.

Archimbaud JP, Banssillon VG, Bernhardt JP, Revillard JP, Perrin J, Traeger J, Carraz M, Fries D, Saubier EC, Bonnet P, Brochier J, Zech P (1969). Technique, surveillance and value of the drainage of the thoracic duct, executed in view of a renal transplantation. J Chir 98(3):211-230.

Baldamus CA, McKenzie IFC, Winn HJ, Russell PS (1973). Acute destruction by humoral antibody of rat skin grafted to mice. J Immunol 110(6):1532-1541.

Barber WH, Mankin JA, Laskow DA, Dierhoi MH, Julian BA, Curtis JJ, Diethelm AG (1991). Long term results of a controlled prospective study with transfusion of donor-specific bone marrow in 56 cadaveric renal allograft recipients. Transplantation 51:70-75.

Bier M, Beavers CD, Merriman WG, Merkel FK, Eiseman B, Starzl TE (1970). Selective plasmapheresis in dogs for delay of heterograft response. Transactions—Trans Am Soc Art Intern Organs 16:325-333.

Bird G, Friend P, Donaldson P, O'Grady J, Portmann B, Calne R, Williams R (1989). Hyperacute rejection in liver transplantation. A case report. Transplant Proc 21:3742-3744.

Brendel W, Duswald KH, von Scheel J, Chaussy C, Sollinger HW, Hammer C (1977). Prolonged survival time of canine xenografts using a new schedule of horse anti-dog lymphocyte globulin (ALG) therapy. Transplant Proc. 9(1):379-381.

Calne RY, White HJO, Yoffa DE, Maginn RR, Binns RM, Samuel JR, Molina VP (1967a). Observation of orthotopic liver transplantation in the pig. Br Med J, 2(550):478-480.

Calne RY, White JHO, Yoffa DE, Binns RM, Maginn RR, Herbertson RM, Millard PR, Molina VP, Davies DR (1967b). Prolonged survival of liver transplants in the pig. Br Med J, 4(500):645-648.

Calne RY, White HJO, Binns RM, Herbertson RM, Millard PR, Pena J, Salman JR, Samuel JR, Davies DR (1969). Immunosuppressive effects of the orthotopically transplanted porcine liver. Transplant Proc, 1(1):321-324.

Calne RY, Davis DR, Pena JR, Balner H, De Vries M, Herberston BM, Joysey VC, Millard PR, Seaman MJ, Samuel JR, Stibbe J, Westbroeck DL (1970a). Hepatic allografts and xenografts in primates. Lancet 1(683):103-106, Jan. 17.

Calne RY (1970b). Organ transplantation between widely disparate species. Transplant Proc, 2(4):550-556.

Cardella CJ, Sutton D, Uldall PR, DeVeber GA (1977). Intensive plasma exchange and renal transplant rejection. Lancet 1(8005):264.

Caridis DT, Liegeois A, Barrett I, Monaco AP (1973). Enhanced survival of canine renal allografts of ALS-treated dogs given bone marrow. Transplant Proc 5:671-674.

Clark DS, Gewurz H, Good RA, Varco RL (1964). Complement fixation during homograft rejection. Surg Forum 15:144-146.

Clark DS, Foker JE, Pickering R, Good RA, Varco RL (1966). Evidence for two platelet populations in xenograft rejection. Surg Forum 17:264-266.

Cordier G, Carnier H, Clot JP, Clampez P, Gorin JP, Clot P, Rassinier JP, Nizza M, Levy R (1966). Orthotopic liver graft in pigs. 1st results. Mem Del Acad De Chir, 92(27):799-807.

Davies HS, Pollard SG, Calne RY (1989). Soluble HLA antigens in the circulation of liver graft recipients. Transplantation, 47:524-527.

Demetris AJ, Jaffe J, Tzakis A, Ramsey G, Todo S, Belle S, Esquivel C, Shapiro R, Markus B, Mrozec E, Van Thiel DH, Sysnl T, Gordon R, Makowka L, Starzl TE (1988). Antibody mediated rejection of human orthotopic liver allografts: A study of liver transplantation across ABO blood group barriers. Am J Pathol, 132:489-502.

Demetris AJ, Jaffe R, Tzakis A, Ramsey G, Todo S, Belle S, Esquivel C, Shapiro R, Zajko A, Markus B, Morozec E, Van Thiel DH, Sysyn G, Gordon R, Makowka L, Starzl TE (1989). Antibody mediated rejection of human liver allografts: Transplantation across ABO Blood group barriers. Transplant Proc 21 (Suppl.1): 2217-2220.

Demetris AJ, Murase N, Nakamura K, Iwaki Y, Yagihashi A, Valdivia L, Todo S, Iwatsuki S, Takaya S, Fung JJ, Starzl TE (1992). Immunopathology of antibodies as effectors of orthotopic liver allograft rejection. Semin Liver Dis 12(1):51-59.

Eichwald EJ, Bernhard AJ, Jorgensen C (1985). Cell-mediated hyperacute rejection. VIII. The recipient's role in adoptive transfer. Transplantation 39(2):219-220.

Estevam Ianhez L, Verginelli G, Sabbaga E, Campos Freire JG (1974). Thoracic duct drainage in human kidney allotransplantation. Revista Brasileira De Pesquisas Medicas E Biologicas 7(3):265-272.

First RM (1992). Transplantation in the nineties. Transplantation 53(1):1-11.

Fischel RJ, Ascher NL, Payne WD, Freese DK, Stack P, Fasola C, Najarian JS (1989). Pediatric liver transplantation across ABO blood group barriers. Transplant Proc 21:2221-2222.

Fischel RJ, Bolman RM III, Platt JL, Najariam JS, Bach FH, Matas AJ (1990). Removal of IgM anti-endothelial antibodies results in prolonged cardiac xenograft survival. Transplant Proc, 22(3):1077-1078.

Flye MW, Duffy BF, Phelan DL, Ratner LE, Mohanakumar T (1990). Protective effects of liver transplantation on a simultaneously transplanted kidney in a highly sensitized patient. Transplantation 50(6):1051-1054.

Forbes RDC, Guttman RD (1982). Evidence for complement induced endothelial injury in vivo. Am J Path, 106(3):378-387.

Forbes RDC, Guttman RD (1984). Pathogenetic studies of cardiac allograft rejection using inbred rat models. Immunological Reviews, 77:5-29.

Forsgren A, Sjoguist J (1966). "Protein A" from S. aureus. J Immunol 97:822-827.

Franksoon C, Blomstrand R (1967). Drainage of the thoracic lymph duct during homologous kidney transplantation in man. Scand J Urol Nephrol 1:123-131.

Franksson C (1964). Letter to the editor. Survival of homografts of skin in rats depleted of lymphocytes by chronic drainage from the thoracic duct. Lancet 1:1331-1332.

Franksson C, Lungre G, Magnusson G, Ringden O

(1976). Drainage of thoracic duct lymph in renal transplant patients. Transplantation 21:133-140.

Fung J, Makowka L, Tzakis A, Klintmalm G, Duquesnoy R, Gordon R, Todo S, Griffin M, Starzl TE (1988). Combined liver-kidney transplantation: Analysis of patients with preformed lymphocytotoxic antibodies. Transplant Proc 20(Suppl. 1):88-91.

Furuya T, Murase N, Demetris AJ, Todo S, Woo J, Starzl TE. (1993) The effect of lymphocytotoxic antibodies after skin, heart or blood sensitization on allograft survival: A comparison of heart and liver. Hepatology (in press).

Gambiez L, Weill BT, Chereau CH, Calmus Y, Houmin D (1990). The hyperacute rejection of guinea pig to rat heart xenografts is mediated by preformed IgM. Transplant Proc, 22(3):1058.

Garnier H, Clot JP, Bertrand M, Camplez P, Kunlin A, Gorin JP, Le Goaziou F, Levy R, Cordier G (1965). Greffe de foie chez le porc; Approache chirurgical. C R. Acad Sci 260:5621-5623.

Garnier H, Clot JP, Chomette G. (1970) Orthotopic transplantation of the porcine liver. Surg Gynecol Obstet, 130(1):105-111.

Gerwurz H, Clark DS, Finstad J, Kelley WD, Varco RL, Good Ra, Gabrielson AE (1966). Role of C' in graft rejection in experimental animals and man. Ann NY Acad Sci 129:673-713.

Giles GR, Boehmig JH, Lilly J, Amemiya H, Takagi H, Coburg AJ, Hathaway WE, Wilson CB, Dixon FJ, Starzl TE (1970). Mechanism and modification of rejection of heterografts between divergent species. Transplant Proc, 2:522-537.

Gjorstrup P (1988). Presentation given at a conference on immunoadsorption sponsored by E.I. DuPont de Nemours and Company, September.

Gordon RD, Iwatsuki S, Esquivel CO, Tzakis A, Todo S, Starzl TE (1986a). Liver transplantation across ABO Blood groups. Surgery, 100:342-348.

Gordon RD, Fung JJ, Markus B, Fox I, Iwatsuki S, Esquivel CO, Tzakis A, Todo S, Starzl TE (1986b). The antibody crossmatch in liver transplantation. 100:705-715.

Gubernatis G, Lauchart W, Jonker M, Steinhoff G, Bornscheuer A, Neuhaus P, van Es AA, Kemnitz J, Wonigeit K, Pichlmayr R (1987).

Signs of hyperacute rejection of liver grafts in rhesus monkeys after donor-specific presensitization. Transplant Proc, 19:1082-1083.

Gugenheim J, Houssin D, Emond J, Gigou M, Crougneau S, Bismuth H (1985). Delayed rejection of heart allografts in hypersensitized rats by extra corporeal donor-specific liver transplantation. Transplantation 41(3):398-400.

Gugenheim J, Charpentier B, Gigou M, Cuomo O, Calise F, Amorosa L, Astarcioglu I, Trias I, Folch M, Martin B, Bismuth H (1988a). Delayed rejection of heart allografts after extracorporeal donor specific liver hemoperfusion. Transplantation 45:628-632.

Gugenheim J, Le Thai B, Rouger P, Gigou M, Gane P, Vial MC, Charpentier B, Reynes M, Bismuth H (1988b). Relationship between the liver and lymphocytotoxic alloantibodies in inbred rats. Transplantation, 45:474-478.

Gugenheim J, Samuel D, Fabiani B, Saliba F, Castaing D, Reynes M, Bismuth H (1989). Rejection of ABO incompatible liver allografts in man. Transplant Proc 21:2223-2224.

Gugenheim J, Samuel D, Reynes M, Bismuth H (1990). Liver transplantation across ABO blood group barriers. Lancet 336:519-523.

Hanto DW, Snover DC, Sibley RK, Noreen HJ, Gajl-Pezalska KJ, Najarian JS, Ascher NL (1987). Hyperacute rejection of a human orthotopic liver allograft in a presensitized recipient. Clin Transplant 1:304-310.

Hasan R, Van den Bogaerde J, Forty J, Wright L, Wallwork J, White DJ (1992). Xenograft adaptation is dependent on the presence of antispecies antibody, not prolonged residence in the recipient. Transplant Proc 24(2):531-532, 1992.

Hawkins E, Mammen E, Rosenberg JC (1971). Effects of heparin and steroids on hyperacutely rejected renal xenografts. J Surg Res 11(10):492-495.

Houssin D, Gugenheim J, Bellon B, Brunaud MD, Gigou M, Charra M, Crougneau S, Bismuth H (1985). Absence of hyperacute rejection of liver allografts in hypersensitized rats. Transplant Proc, 17:293-295.

Houssin D, Bellon B, Brunaud MD, Gugenheim J, Settaf A, Meriggi F, Emond J (1986). Interactions between liver allografts and lymphocytotoxic alloantibodies in inbred rats. Hepatology 6(5):994-998.

Hume DM, Williams GM (1969). Personal communication, February 8, 1969. Cited in Starzl TE: Experience in hepatic transplantation, W.B. Saunders, Philadelphia, p.269.

Ildstad ST, Wren SM, Barbieri SA, Sachs DH (1985). Characterization of mixed allogeneic chimeras: Immunocompetence, in vitro reactivity, and genetic specificity of tolerance. J Exp Med 162:231-244.

Inamura H, Hashimoto M, Nakahara K, Aoki H, Yamaguchi I, Kohsaka M (1988). Immunosuppressive effect of FK506 on collagen-induced arthritis in rats. Clin Immunol Immunopathol 46(1):82-90

Iwaki Y, Lau M, Terasaki PI (1988). Successful transplants across T warm-positive crossmatches due to IgM antibodies. Clin Transpl 2(2):81-84.

Iwaki Y, Starzl TE, Yagihashi A, Taniwaki S, Abu-Elmagd K, Tzakis A, Fung J, Todo S (1991). Replacement of donor lymphoid tissue in human small bowel transplants under FK 506 immunosuppression. Lancet 337:818-819.

Iwatsuki S, Iwaki Y, Kano T, Klintmalm G, Koep LJ, Weil R, Starzl TE (1981). Successful liver transplantation from crossmatch-positive donors. Transplant Proc, 13:286-288.

Iwatsuki S, Rabin BS, Shaw BW Jr, Starzl TE (1984). Liver transplantation against T Cell-positive warm crossmatches. Transplant Proc, 16:1427-1429.

Johnson HK, Niblack GD, Tallent MB, Richie RE (1977). Immunologic preparation for cadaver renal transplant by thoracic duct drainage. Transplantation Proc 9:1499-1503.

Johnston PS, Wang MW, Lim SM, Wright LS, Wite DJ (1992). Discordant xenograft rejection in an antibody-free model. Transplantation, 54(4):573-576.

Kamada N (1988). Experimental liver transplantation. CRC Press, Inc, Boca Raton, Florida.

Karuppan S, Ericzon BG, Moller E (1991). Relevance of a positive crossmatch in liver transplantation. Transplant Int 4:18-25.

Kemp E, Kemp G, Svendsen P, Nielsen E, Buhl MR (1976). Prolongation of xenograft survival by infusion of heterologous antibodies against recipient serum. Acta Pathol Microbiol Scand 84(4):342-344.

Kemp E, Kemp G, Abildgard-Jacobsen I, Lundborg C (1977). Prolongation of survival of renal xenografts by infusion of donor blood. Acta Pathol Microbiol Scand (a), 85A(2):267-269.

Kemp E, Kemp G, Starklint H, Larsen S (1982). Immunosuppression with cobra venom factor, anti-platelet aggregator, and cyclosporin A in renal xenotransplantation. Transplant Proc, 14:11-118.

Kemp E, Steinbruchel D, Starklint H, Larsen S, Henriksen I, Dieperink H (1987). Renal xenograft rejection: Prolonging effect of captopril, ACE-inhibitors, prostacyclin, and cobra venom factor. Transplant Proc 19(6):4471-4474.

Kemp E, White D, Dieperink H, Larsen S, Starklint H, Steinbruchel D (1987a). Delayed rejection of rabbit kidneys transplanted into baby pigs. Transplant Proc, 19(1 pt 2):1143-1144.

Kino T, Hatanaka H, Hashimoto M, Nishiyana N, Goto T, Okuhara M, Kohsaka M, Aoki H, Imanaka H (1987b). FK 506, a novel immunosuppressant isolated from a streptomyces I. Fermentation, isolation, and physico chemical and biological characteristics. J Antibiot (Tokyo) 40(9):1249-1255.

Kirubakaran MG, Disney APS, Norman J, Pugsley DJ, Mathew TH (1981). Trial of plasmapheresis in the treatment of renal allograft rejection. Transplantation 32:164-165.

Kissmeyer-Nielsen F, Olsen S, Petersen VP, Fjeldborg O (1966). Hyperacute rejection of kidney allografts associated with pre-existing humoral antibodies against donor cells. Lancet, 2:662-665.

Knechtle SJ, Kolbeck PC, Tsuchimoto S, Coundouriotis A, Sanfilippo F, Bollinger RR (1987a). Hepatic transplantation into sensitized recipients. Demonstration of hyperacute rejection. Transplantation, 43(1):8-12.

Knechtle SJ, Kolbeck PC, Tsuchimoto S, Coundouriotis A, Sanfilippo F, Bollinger RR (1987b). Experimental liver transplantation. Transplant Proc, 19:1072-1076.

Koep LJ, Weill III R, Starzl TE (1980). The technique of prolonged thoracic duct drainage in transplantation. Surg Gynecol Obstet 151:61-64.

Kux M, Boehmig HJ, Amemiya H, Torisu M, Yokoyama T, Launois B, Popovtzer MM, Wilson CB, Dixon FJ, Starzl TE (1971). Modification of hyperacute canine renal homograft and pig-to-dog heterograft rejection by the intra-arterial infusion of citrate. Surgery 70:103-112.

Landsteiner K (1962). Specificity of Serological Reactions. New York: Dover (Publisher).

Lempinen G, Salmenkivik K, Sivula A (1971). Orthotopic liver transplantation in the pig. Acta Chir Scand, 137(3):265-270.

Makowka L, Miller C, ChapChap P, Podesta L, Pan C, Pressley D, Mazzaferro V, Esquivel CO, Todo S, Banner B, Jaffe R, Saunders R, Starzl TE (1987). Prolongation of pig-to-dog renal xenograft survival by modification of the in-flammatory mediator response. Ann Surg, 206:482-495.

Marino IR, Weber T, Esquivel CO, Kang YG, Starzl TE, Duquesnoy RJ (1988). Intra-operative blood transfusion requirements and deficient hemostasis in highly alloimmunized patients undergoing liver transplantation. Transplant Proc 20(6):1087-1089.

Marino IR, Ferla G, Celli S, Stieber A, Muttillo I, Maggiano N, Perrelli L, Musiani P (1990). Hyperacute rejection of renal discordant xe-nograft (pig-to-rabbit): Model assessment and rejection mechanisms. Transplant Proc, 22(3):1071-1076.

Marino IR, Celli S, Ferla G, Stieber AC, Maggiano N, Musiani P (1991). Histopathological, immun-ofluorescent, and electron-microscopic features of hyperacute rejection in discordant renal xe-notransplantation. In: Xenotransplantation, Coop DKC, Kemp E, Reemtsma K, White DJG (eds), pp. 207-230, Springer-Verlag, Ber-lin.

Marino IR, Doyle HR (1993). Conventional Im-munosuppressive Drugs In: Immunosuppres-sive Drugs: Advances in Anti-Rejection Therapy. Thomson AW, Starzl TE (Eds). Edward Arnold, Publishers (in press)

Marquet FL, van Es AA, Heystek GA, van Leersum RH, Balner H (1978). Prolongation of ba-boon to rhesus kidney xenograft survival by pretransplant rhesus blood transfusions. Transplantation 25(3):165-166.

Martelli A, Bonomini V (1970). In: Bertelli A, Monaco AP (eds). Pharmacological treatment in organ and tissue transplantation. Balti-more: Williams & Wilkins, 140.

Mazzoni G, Martino CD, Melis M, Demofonti A,

Valli A, Francesconi M, Pellegrini S (1971). Organ transplantation in pig with different portal and caval venous drainage. Eur Surg Res, 3(1):62-71.

Merkel FK, Bier M, Beavers DC, Merriman WG, Wilson C, Starzl TE (1971). Modification of xenograft response by selective plasma-pheresis. Transplant Proc 3:534-537.

Moberg AW, Shoms AR, Gewurz H, Moze M, Najarian JS (1971). Prolongation of renal xenografts by the simultaneous sequestration of preformed antibody, inhibition of comple-ment, coagulation and antibody synthesis. Transplant Proc 3(1):538-541.

Monaco AP, Wood ML (1970). Studies on heterolo-gous antilymphocyte serum in mice: VII. Op-timal cellular antigen for induction of immu-nologic tolerance with ALS. Transplant Proc 2(4):489-496.

Moran M, Mozes MF, Maddux MS, Veremis S, Bartkus C, Ketel B, Pollak R, Wallemark C, Jonasson O (1990). Prevention of acute graft rejection by the prostaglandin E1 analogue misoprostol in renal-transplant recipients treated with cyclosporine and prednisone. New Engl J Med 322:1183-1188.

Mundy AR (1980). Prolongation of cat to dog renal xenograft survival with prostacyclin. Trans-plantation 30:226-228.

Murase N, Starzl TE, Demetris AJ, Valdivia L, Tanabe M, Cramer D, Makowka L (1993). Hamster to rat heart and liver xenotransplan-tation with FK506 plus antiproliferative drugs. Transplantation (in press)

Murray JE, Wilson RE, Tilney NL, Merrill JP, Cooper WC, Birtch AG, Carpenter CB, Hager EB, Dammin GJ, Harrison JH (1968). Five years' experience in renal transplantation with immunosuppressive drugs: Survival, func-tion, complications, and the role of lympho-cyte depletion by thoracic duct fistula. Ann Surg 168:416-435.

Naik RB, Ashlin R, Wilson C, Smith DS, Lee HA, Slapak M (1979). The role of plasmapheresis in renal transplantation. Clin Nephrol 5:245-250.

Nakamura K, Yagihashi A, Iwaki Y, Takaya S, Hartman GG, Murase N, Bronsther O, Manez R, Fung JJ, Iwatsuki S, Starzl TE, Demetris AJ (1991). The lymphocytotoxic crossmatch in liver transplantation: A clinicopathologic analysis. Transplant Proc 23:3021-3022.

Ohshima S, Ono Y, Kinukawa T, Matsuura O, Takeuchi N, Hattori R (1987). The beneficial effects of thoracic duct drainage in HLA-1 haplotype identical kidney transplantation. J Urol 138(1):33-35.

Ohshima S, Ono Y, Kinukawa T, Matsuura O, Takeuchi N, Hirabayashi S (1988). The beneficial effect of thoracic duct drainage pretreatment in living related kidney transplantation. Transplant Proc 20:415.

Ohshima S, Ono Y, Kinukawa T, Matsuura O, Takeuchi N, Hattori R (1989). The long-term results of thoracic duct drainage in living related kidney transplantation. Transplantation Proc 21:1972-1973.

Ono Y, Ohshima S, Kinukawa T, Matsuura O, Hirabayashi S (1987). MLR suppression and MLR-suppressor activity induced by thoracic duct drainage prior to transplantation. Transplant Proc 19(1 Pt 3):1985-1987.

Orosz CG, Zinn NE, Sirinek LP, Ferguson RM (1986). Delayed rejection of heart allografts in hypersensitized rats by extracorporeal donor specific liver hemoperfusion. Transplantation, 41:398-404.

Palmer A, Taube D, Welsh K, Bewick M, Gjorstrup P, Thick M (1987). Removal of anti-HLA antibodies: Preliminary clinical experience. Transplant Proc 19:3750-3751.

Palmer A, Taube D, Welsh K, Bewick M, Gjorstrup P, Thick M (1989). Removal of anti-HLA antibodies by extracorporeal immunoadsorption to enable renal transplantation. Lancet 1:10-12.

Peacock JH and Terblanche J (1967). Orthotopic homotransplantation of the liver in the pig. In: The Liver, Read AE (Ed), Butterworths, London, 333-336.

Perper RJ, Najarian JS (1966a). Experimental renal heterotransplantation. I. In widely divergent species. Transplantation, 4(4):700-712.

Perper RJ, Najarian JS (1966b). Experimental renal heterotransplantation: II. Closely related species. Transplantation, 4(6):700-712.

Power D, Nicholls A, Muirhead N, MacLeod AM, Engeset J, Catta GR, Edward N (1981). Plasma exchange in acute renal allograft rejection: Is a controlled trial really necessary? Transplantation 32(2):162-163.

Quagliata F, Lawrence VJW, Phillips-Quagliata JM (1972). Short communication: Prostag-landin E as a regulator of lymphocyte function selective action on B lymphocytes and synergy with procerbasine in digression of immune responses. Cellular Immunol 6:457-465.

Rappaport RS, Dodge GR (1982). Prostaglandin E inhibits the production of human Interleukin 2. J Exp Med 155:943-949.

Rego J, Prevost F, Rumeau JL, Modesto A, Fourtanier G, Durand D, Suc JM, Ohayon E, Ducos J (1987). Hyperacute rejection after ABO incompatible orthotopic liver transplantation. Transplant Proc 19:4589-4590.

Rifle G, Chalopin JM, Turc JM, Guigner F, Vialtel P, Dechelette E, Chenais F, Cordonnier D (1979). Plasmapheresis in the treatment of renal allograft rejections. Transplant Proc 11(1):20-26.

Rose AG (1991). Histopathology of Cardiac Xenograft Rejection. In: Xenotransplantation: The Transplantation of Organs and Tissues Between Species. Cooper DKC, Kemp E, Reemtsma K, White DJG (Eds), Springer-Verlag Publishers, Berlin, 13:231-242.

Rosenberg JC, Broersma RJ, Bullemer G, Mammen EF, Lenaghan R, Rosenberg BF (1969). Relationship of platelets, blood coagulation, and fibrinolysis to hyperactue rejection of renal xenografts. Transplantation 8(2):152-161.

Rosenberg JC, Hawkins E, Mammen E, Palutke M, Riddle J, Rosenberg BF (1971a). Hyperacute rejection of heterografts: Studies of pig to dog renal transplants. In: Von Kaulla K, Thomas CC (eds), Coagulation Problems in Transplanted Organs.

Rosenberg JC, Hawkins E, Rector F (1971b). Mechanisms of immunological injury during antibody-mediated hyperacute rejection of renal heterografts. Transplantation 11(2):151-157.

Sanchez-Urdazpal L, Sterioff S, Janes C, Schwerman L, Rosen C, Krom RA (1991). Increased bile duct complications in ABO incompatible liver transplant recipients. Transplant Proc 23:1440-1441.

Sarles HE, Remmers Jr AR, Fish JC, Canales CO, Thomas FD, Tyson DR, Beathard GA, Ritzmann SE (1970). Depletion of lymphocytes for the protection of renal allografts. Arch Intern Med 125:443-450.

Shapiro R, Scantlebury V, Tzakis AG, Makowka L,

Watt R, Oks A, Yanaga K, Podesta L, Casavilla A, Wos S, Murray J, Oral A, D'Andrea P, Banner B, Starzl TE (1990a). Immuno-depletion in xenotransplantation. J Invest Surg 3:39-49.

Shapiro R, Starzl TE (1990b). Renal transplantation in the highly sensitized patient: The role of thoracic duct drainage, plasmapheresis, and staph A immunodepletion. Therapeutic Plasmapheresis, T. Ota (Ed), Tokoyo, 8:13-24.

Shaw JRL (1985). Role of prostaglandins in transplantation. In: Cohen MM ed. Biological Protection with Prostaglandins. Vol 1, Boca Raton: CRC Press Inc. 111-128.

Shons AR, Jetzer J, Moberg AW, Najarian JS. (1970). Prolongation of heterograft survival by electrophoretic extraction of preformed antibody. Surg Forum 21:263.

Shons AR, Bier M, Jetzer T, Najarian JS (1973). Techniques of in vivo plasma modification for the treatment of hyperacute rejection. Surg 73(1):28-37.

Shons AR, Najarian JS (1974a). Xenograft rejection mechanisms in man. Trans Am Soc Artif Intern Organs 20:B562-B568.

Shons AR, Najarian JS (1974b). Modification of xenograft rejection by aspirin, dextran, and cinanserin: The importance of platelets in hyperacute rejection. Transplant Proc 6(4):435-440.

Slavin S, Strober S, Fuks Z, Kaplan HS (1977). Induction of specific tissue transplantation tolerance using fractionated total lymphoid irradiation in adult mice: Long-term survival of allogeneic bone marrow and skin grafts. J. Exp Med 146:34-48.

Sonoda T, Takaha M, Kusunoki T (1966). Prolonged thoracic duct lymph drainage. Application for human renal homotransplantation. Arch Surg 93:831-833.

Starzl TE (1964). Experience In Renal Transplantation. WB Saunders Company, Philadelphia, PA.

Starzl TE. Experience in Hepatic Transplantation, WB Saunders, Philadelphia, 1969.

Starzl TE, Boehmig HJ, Amemiya H, Wilson CB, Dixon FJ, Giles GR, Simpson KM, Halgrimson CG (1970). Clotting changes including disseminated intravascular coagulation, during rapid renal-homograft rejection. New Engl J

Med 283:383-390.

Starzl TE, Ishikawa M, Putnam CW, Porter KA, Picache R, Husberg BS, Halgrimson CG, Schroter G (1974). Progress in and deterrents to orthotopic liver transplantation, with special reference to survival, resistance to hyperacute rejection, and biliary duct reconstruction. Transplant Proc, 6:129-139.

Starzl TE, Koep LJ, Weill III R, Halgrimson CG, Franks JJ (1979a). Thoracic duct drainage in organ transplantation: Will it permit better immunosuppression? Transplantation Proc 11;276-284.

Starzl TE, Weill III R, Koep LJ, McCalmon RT, Terasaki PI, Iwaki Y, Schroter GPJ, Franks JJ, Subryan BS, Halgrimson CG (1979b). Thoracic duct fistula and renal transplantation. Ann Surg 190:474-486.

Starzl TE, Weill III R, Koep LJ, Iwaki Y, Teraski PI, Schroter PJ (1979c). Thoracic duct drainage before and after cadaveric kidney transplantation. Surg Gynecol Obstet 149:815-821.

Starzl TE, Weill III R, Koep LJ (1979D). The pretreatment principle in renal transplantation as illustrated by thoracic duct drainage. Presented in part at the Dialysis and Kidney Transplantation 25th Anniversary Celebration, Boston, Massachusetts, September 15.

Starzl TE, Klintmalm GBG, Iwatsuki S, Schroter G, Weill III R (1981). Late follow-up after thoracic duct drainage in cadaveric renal transplantation. Surg Gynecol Obstet 153:377-382

Starzl TE, Tzakis A, Makowka L, Banner B, Demetris A, Ramsey G, Duquesnoy R, Griffin M (1987). The definition of ABO factors in transplantation: Relation to other humoral antibody states. Transplant Proc, 19:4492-4497.

Starzl TE, Demetris AJ, Todo S, Kang Y, Tzakis A, Duquesnoy R, Makowka L, Banner B, Concepcion W, Porter KA (1989). Evidence for hyperacute rejection of human liver grafts: The case of the carnary kidneys. Clin Transplant 3(1):37-45.

Starzl TE, Demetris A (submitted). The HLA matching controversy. New Engl J Med.

Starzl TE, Fung J, Tzakis A, Todo S, Demetris AJ, Marino IR, Doyle H, Zeevi A, Warty V, Michaels M, Kusne S, Rudert WA, Trucco M (1993). Baboon to human liver transplantation. Lancet 341 (8837):65-71.

Starzl TE, Thomson AW, Todo S, Fung JJ (1991). First International Congress on FK506. Transplant Proc 23(6):2709-3380.

Strom TB, Carpenter CB (1983). Prostaglandin as an effective antirejection therapy in rat renal allograft recipients. Transplantation 35:279-281.

Suminoto R, Shinomiya T (1991). Examination of serum class I antigen in liver transplanted rats. Clin Exp Immunol, 85:114-120.

Takagishi K, Kaibara N, Hotokebuchi T, Arita C, Morinaga M, Arai K (1985). Serum transfer of collagen arthritis in congenitally athymic nude rats. J Immunol 134(6):3864-3867.

Takagishi K, Yamamoto M, Nishimura A, Yamasaki G, Kanazawa N, Hotokebuchi T, Kaibara N (1989). Effects of FK 506 on collegan arithritis in mice. Transplant Proc 21(1):1053-1055.

Takaya S, Duquesnoy R, Iwaki Y, Demetris J, Yagihashi A, Bronsther O, Iwatsuki S, Starzl TE (1991). Positive crossmatch in primary human liver allografts under cyclosporine of FK 506 therapy. Transplant Proc 23:396-399.

Takaya S, Bronsther O, Iwaki Y, Nakamura K, Abu-Elmagd K, Yagihashi A, Demetris JA, Kobayashi M, Todo S, Tzakis A, Fung JJ, Starzl TE (1992a). The adverse impact on liver transplantation of using positive cytotoxic crossmatch donors. Transplantation 53:400-406

Takaya S, Iwaki Y, Starzl TE (1992b). Liver transplantation in positive cytotoxic crossmatch cases using FK506, high dose steroids and prostaglandin E1. Transplantation 54:927-930.

Taube DH, Welsh KI, Kennedy LA, Thick MG, Bewick M, Cameron JS, Ogg CS, Rudge CJ, Williams DG (1984a). Successful removal and prevention of resynthesis of anti-HLA antibody. Transplantation 37(3):254-255.

Taube DH, Williams DG, Cameron JS, Bewick M, Ogg CS, Rudge CJ, Welsh KI, Kennedy LA, Thick MG (1984b). Renal transplantation after removal and prevention of resynthesis of HLA antibodies. Lancet 1(8381):824-828.

Terasaki PI, Marchioro TL, Starzl TE (1965). Serotyping of human lymphocyte antigens. Preliminary trials on long-term kidney homograft survivors. In: Histocompatibility Testing National Acad Sci-National Res Council, Washington DC, pp. 83-96.

Thomas J, Carver M, Foil B, Haisch C, Thomas F (1983). Renal allograft tolerance induced with ATG and donor bone marrow in outbred rhesus monkeys. Transplantation 36:104-106.

Tilney NL, Murray JE (1968). Chronic thoracic duct fistula: Operative technique and physiologic effects in man. Ann Surg 167:1-8.

Tilney NL, Atkinson JC, Murray JE (1970). The immunosuppressive effect of thoracic duct drainage in human kidney transplantation. Ann Intern Med 72:59-64.

Valdivia LA, Mondem M, Gotoh M, Hasuike Y, Kubota N, Emdoh W, Okamura J, Mori T (1987a). Hepatic xenografts from hamster-to-rat. Transplant Proc, 19(1 of 2):1158-1159.

Valdivia LA, Monden M, Gotoh M, Hasuike Y, Kubota N, Ichikawa T, Okamura J, Mori T (1987b). Prolonged survival of hamster-to-rat liver xenografts using splenectomy and cyclosporine administration. Transplantation 44:759-763.

Walker WE, Niblack GD, Richie RE, Johnson HK, Tallent MB (1977). Use of thoracic duct drainage in human renal transplantation. Surg Forum 28:316-317.

Williams GM, Hume DM, Hudson RP Jr, Morris PJ, Kano K, Milgrom F (1968). "Hyperacute" renal-homograft rejection in man. New Engl J Med, 279(12):611-618.

Winn HJ, Baldamus CA, Jooste SV, Russell PS (1973). Acute destruction by humoral antibody of rat skin grafted to mice. J Exp Med 137(4):893-910.

Woo J, Stephen M, Thomson AW (1988). Spleen lymphocyte populations and expression of activation markers in rats treated with the potent new immunosuppressive agent FK506. Immunolgy 65:153-155.

Woodle ES, Perorizet GA, Brunt EM, So SKS, Jendrisak MD, McCullough CS, Vehe KL, White HM, Peters MG, Marsh JW (1991). FK506: Reversal of humorally mediated rejection following ABO-incompatible liver transplantation. Transplant Proc 23(6):2992-2993.

INDEX